CLINICAL MEDICINE
Self-Assessment Questions in Colour

Pierre-Marc G Bouloux BSc, MD, FRCP

Senior Lecturer in Endocrinology
Academic Department of Medicine
Royal Free Hospital
London UK

M WOLFE

St. Louis Baltimore Boston Chicago London Philadelphia Sydney Toronto

ISBN 1-56375-613-7

Cataloguing in Publication Data
CIP catalogue records for this book are available from the British Library and
the US Library of Congress.

Publisher:	Michele Campbell
Project managers:	Stephen McGrath
	Moira Sarsfield
Design:	Jim Evoy
Production:	Susan Bishop
	Jane Tozer

Originated in Hong Kong by Mandarin Offset.
Printed in Singapore by Imago Productions (FE) Pte Ltd, 1993.

Copyright © 1987 Gower Medical Publishing.
Copyright © 1993 Mosby-Year Book Europe Limited.
Published in 1993 by Wolfe Publishing, an imprint of Mosby-Year Book Europe Limited.
For full details of all Mosby-Year Book Europe Limited titles please write to Mosby-Year
Book Europe Limited, Lynton House, 7–12 Tavistock Square, London,WC1H 9LB,
England.

Preface

The format of each of the twelve chapters of this book follows closely that of a complete MRCP (UK) Part II written examination. Each chapter begins with twenty colour and X-ray/CT/MRI plates, which correspond to the projected material section of the examination. Then follow some case histories of varying length, and a section on interpretation of laboratory data, electrocardiograms, echocardiograms, electrophoretic strips and other investigations. At the end of each chapter there is a list of suggested answers, which are graded 'ideal' (★★★★), 'reasonable' (★★) and 'possible' (★) or in some cases, 'incorrect' (0). The book thus allows a prospective candidate for higher medical training to assess, in a rough and ready way, his or her factual knowledge, observational experience, and interpretive and deductive skill.

This aim alone would perhaps not in itself justify a book of this type. I have set my sights considerably higher.

There are two important respects in which this book is designed also to comprise a short course in postgraduate medicine (although necessarily a somewhat selective one). First, the 'answer' section of each chapter gives in all appropriate cases short explanatory notes which give factual background to the question or questions posed.

Secondly, there is an extensive and complete index at the back of the book which can be used in the same way as the subject index of any medical textbook. For example, under the entry 'Sarcoidosis' there are references to skin and radiological illustrations, laboratory findings, and other clinical information embodied in the explanatory notes for many of the questions.

I trust that undergraduates as well as postgraduate students will find that this book provides them with a way of learning medicine which is complementary to the necessary study of standard texts, and which conveys a little of the excitement, interest and enjoyment of actual medical practice – which starts with the patient rather than with his disease!

In this second edition, I have replaced some of the older material which may be less relevant to current clinical practice, with ultrasonic, echocardiographic, and images from the new radiological modalities such as magnetic resonance imaging with which the student will be expected to be familiar for the examination.

I am indebted to the Department of Medical Illustrations at St. Bartholomew's Hospital for the clinical photographs, Mrs Celia Burrage for invaluable secretarial assistance, and to the staff of Gower Medical Publishing for their skills and perseverance.

P-M G Bouloux

Normal Ranges

Biochemical	SI	Conventional Units
Acid phosphatase	<7.2iu/l	<4KA units/100ml
Alanine amino transferase (ALT)	5–30iu/l	
Albumin	34–48g/l	3.4–4.8g/100ml
Aldosterone – lying, normal diet	135–400pmol/l	48.6–144pg/ml
– standing (4h)	330–830pmol/l	118–298pg/ml
Adrenaline – plasma, supine	<1.0nmol/l	
Alkaline phosphatase	25–100iu/l	3–13.5KA units/100ml
Amylase		<300 Somogyi units
Aspartate aminotransferase (AST)	10–40iu/l	
B12 (serum)	160–900ng/l	
Bicarbonate	22–30mmol/l	22–30mEq/l
Bilirubin	2–17μmol/l	
Calcium	2.2–2.67mmol/l	8.6–10.5mg/100ml
Chloride	95105mmol/l	95–105mEq/l
Cholesterol	3.6–7.8mmol/l	140–303mg/100ml
C3	0.1–0.18g/l	100–180mg/100ml
Copper	14–22μmol/l	17–160μg/100ml
Cortisol 09.00h	170–700nmol/l	6–25μg/100ml
24.00h	<140nmol/l	<5μg/100ml
Creatine phosphokinase (CPK) – male	17–148iu/l	
– female	10–79iu/l	
Creatinine	0.05–0.10mmol/l	0.56–1.13mg/100ml
Folate (serum	4–18μg/l	
Folate (red cell)	160–640μg/l	
Globulin	22–35g/l	2.2–3.5g/100ml
Glucose (fasting)	4.5–5.8mmol/l	80–104mg/100ml
Gamma glutamyl transferase (γGT)	5–30iu/l	
Iron	13–32μmol/l	74–182μg/100ml
Iron binding capacity (TIBC)	40–80μmol/l	

Biochemical	SI	Conventional Units
Lactate	0.6–1.8mmol/l	
Magnesium	0.7–1.1mmol/l	1.4–2.2mg/100ml
Noradrenaline – plasma, supine	0.6–3.1nmol/l	
Oestradiol mid-cycle	500–1100pmol/l	
Osmolality (plasma)	275–295mOsm/kg	
P_aO_2	11.2–14kPa	85–105mmHg
P_aCO_2	4.7–6.0kPa	35–45mmHg
pH	7.35–7.45	
Phosphate	0.8–1.5mmol/l	2.5–4.6mg/100ml
Potassium	3.5–5.0mmol/l	3.5–5.0mEq/l
Prolactin	<360mu/l	<20ng/ml
Protein	62–80g/l	6.2–8.0g/100ml
Renin – lying, normal diet	230–1000pmol/A1/l/h	300–1300pg/ml/h
– standing, (4h)	460–1550pmol/A1/l/h	600–1950pg/ml/h
Salicylate (therapeutic)		<200mg/l
Sex hormone binding globulin (SHBG) – male	15–50nmol/l	
– female	38–103nmol/l	
Sodium	135–146mmol/l	135–146mEq/l
Testosterone – male	9–35nmol/l	
– female	0.9–3.1nmol/l	
Thyroxine	58–174nmol/l	4.6–13.5μg/100ml
Tri-iodothyronine	1.2–3.1nmol/l	
Triglycerides	0.8–2.1mmol/l	40–150mg/dl
Thyroid stimulating hormone (TSH)	0.4–6mu/l	
Urea	2.5–6.7mmol/l	15–40mg/100ml
Uric acid	0.12–0.42mmol/l	2–7mg/100ml

Normal Ranges

Urinary Biochemistry	SI	Conventional Units
Calcium	<7mmol/24h	
Copper	15–78μmol/24h	
Creatinine	9–18mmol/24h	
5 HTAA	5–75μmol/24h	
Metanephrines	<5μmol/25h	
Protein	<0.2g/25h	
Vanillyl mandelic acid (VMA)	5–35μmol/24h	(up to 7mg/25h)

Cerebrospinal Fluid	SI	Conventional Units
Protein	0.15–0.4g/l	15–40mg/100ml
Glucose	2.8–4.5g/l	28–45mg/100ml
Pressure	70–180mmH$_2$O	70–180mmH$_2$O
Cells	0–8 × 10^6/l	0–8/mm^3
Chloride	120–128mmol/l	120–128mEq/l

Haematological	SI	Conventional Units
Haemoglobin – male	13–18g/dl	
– female	11.5–15g/dl	
Red blood cell count – male	4.5–6.5 × 10^{12}/l	4.5–6.5 × 10^6/mm^3
– female	3.9–5.6 × 10^{12}/l	3.9–5.6 × 10^6/mm^3
Haematocrit (PCV) – male	0.4–0.54	
– female	0.35–0.47	
Mean corpuscular Hb (MCH)	27–32pg	27–32μg
Mean corpuscular Hb concentration	32–36g/dl	32–36g/100ml
Mean corpuscular volume (MCV)	76–95fl	76–95μm^3
Platelet count	150–400 × 10^9/l	150–400 × 10^3/mm^3
Reticulocyte count	0.2–2%	
White cell count	4–11 × 10^9/l	4–11 × 10^3/mm^3

Endocrine | SI

ACTH (plasma) 09.00	10–80ng/l
24.00	<10ng/l

Insulin Tolerance test (0.15u/kg) with glucose <2.2mol/l

Peak plasma cortisol	>550nmol/l
Peak serum GH	20–40mU/l

Glucagon test (1mg s.c.)

Peak plasma cortisol	580nmol/l

Short Synacthen test (0.25mg im) at 09.00	mean	95% CT
Plasma cortisol at 30min	820nmol/l	550–1160nmol/l
Plasma cortisol at 60min	990nmol/l	690–1290nmol/l
Increment	580nmol/l	330–850nmol/l

Pituitary Gonadal Function | SI

	SERUM LH (U/l)		SERUM FSH (U/l)	
Female: follicular	2.5–21		1–10	
mid-cycle	25–70		6–25	
luteal	1–13		0.3–2.1	
Male	1–10		1–7	
LHRH test (100µg/iv)	**20min**	**60min**	**20min**	**60min**
Female (follicular)	14–42	12–35	1–11	1–25
Male	13–58	11–48	1–7	1–5

Paper 1

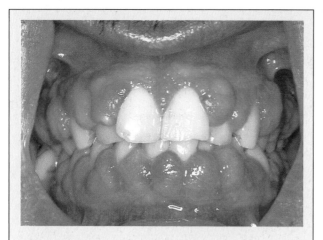

1. This patient was receiving immunosuppressive treatment following a heart transplant.
   (a) What abnormality is shown?
   (b) What is the likely cause?

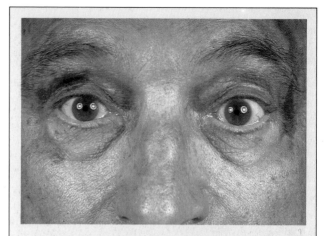

2. This patient presented with heavy proteinuria and complained of spontaneous bruising especially in the face and neck. His ESR was 115mm/h.
   (a) What two abnormalities are shown?
   (b) What is the most likely underlying diagnosis?

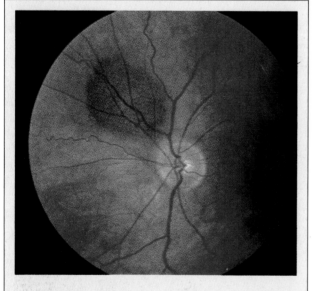

3. This fundal appearance was an incidental finding in a 25-year-old man.
   What is the most likely diagnosis?

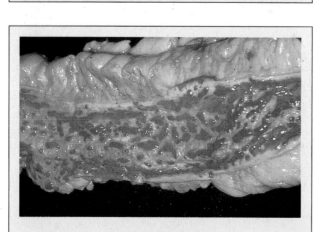

4. This is a segment of colon.
   (a) What is the most likely diagnosis?
   (b) Suggest an alternative diagnosis.

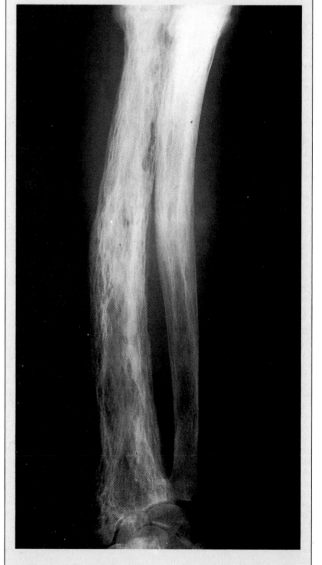

5. What is the diagnosis?

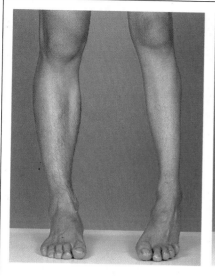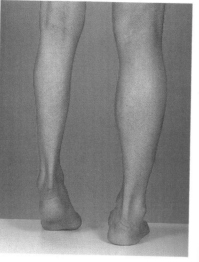

6. What is the likely cause of the appearance of this patient's legs?

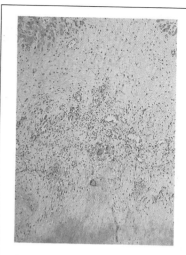

7. This is a section of pericardium, with some heart muscle also visible. What is the diagnosis?

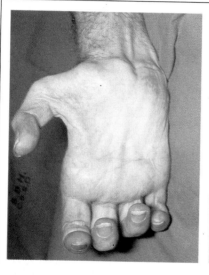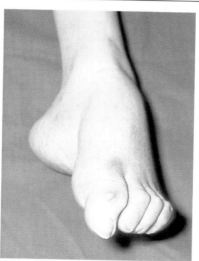

8. List three possible causes of this appearance.

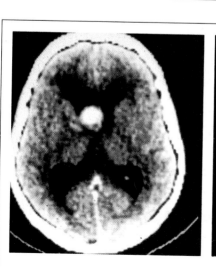

9. This is a CT brain scan with contrast enhancement.
   (a) What two abnormalities are visible?
   (b) What is the likely diagnosis?

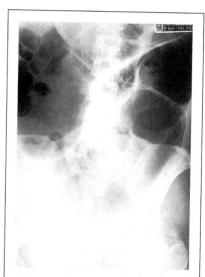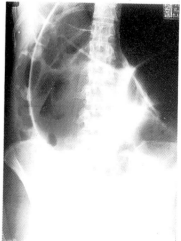

10. These are the supine and erect abdominal radiographs of a 56-year-old woman with abdominal pain and distension of three weeks' duration.
What is the likely diagnosis?

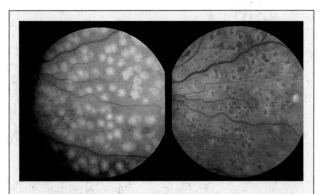

11. What is the cause of these appearances?

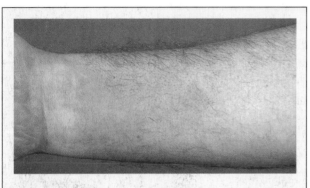

12. This lesion was found on the forearm of a patient taking a laxative.
(a) What is the diagnosis?
(b) Name two drugs with which this lesion is especially associated.

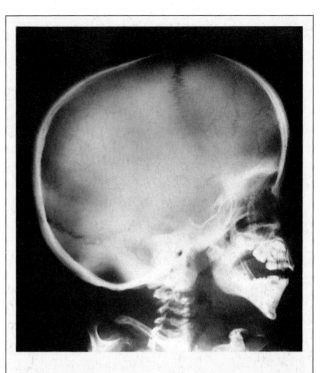

13. What is the diagnosis?

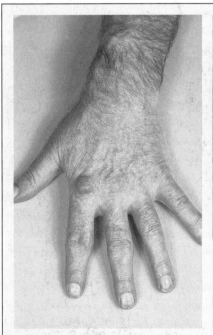

14. (a) What two abnormalities are shown?
(b) What is the probable diagnosis?

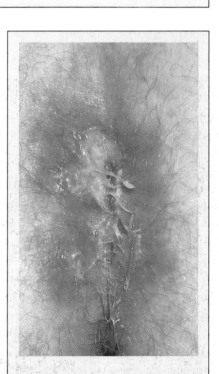

15. This is the perianal region of a patient with the acquired immunodeficiency syndrome (AIDS).
What is the likely cause of the lesion shown?

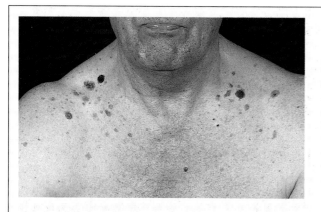 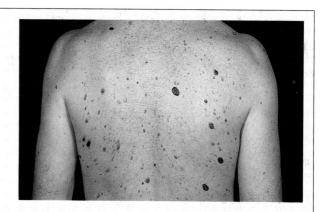

16. This man recently underwent surgery for a colorectal cancer. What is the cause of these multiple lesions on his skin?

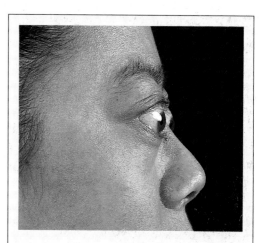

17. What abnormality is shown?

18. What is the most likely cause of this appearance?

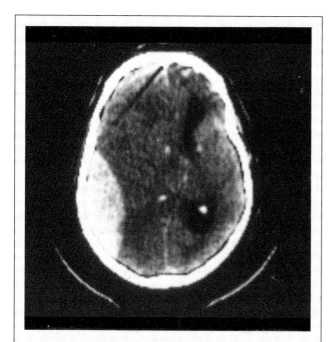

19. This elderly gentleman had sustained a recent head injury. What is the diagnosis?

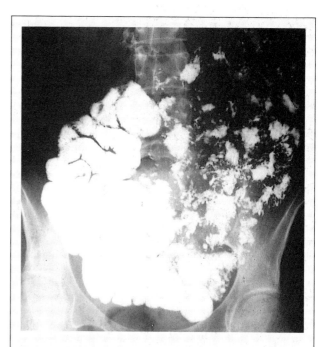

20. This is small bowel enema. What is the diagnosis?

Case Histories

CASE I

A 42-year-old divorcee was admitted to casualty following a bout of vomiting and one small haematemesis. She had suffered depression in the past, and over the previous five years had taken to drinking up to half a bottle of spirits daily. As a result, she had lost her job as a university lecturer.

Three days prior to admission, she had drunk one bottle of vodka over 24 hours. The following day, she had complained of a severe headache and recurrent retching and vomiting. On the day of admission, the vomitus had a 'coffee ground' appearance initially, but the last episode contained almost half a cupful of fresh blood.

On admission she was not shocked, but was clearly distressed. She was unkempt. She was not anaemic, clubbed or jaundiced. Several spider naevi were noted in the upper trunk. The liver was firm and enlarged by 4 cm, but the spleen was not palpable. There was no free fluid in the abdomen. She was given intravenous parenterovite, and began oral cimetidine therapy.

The vomiting subsided, but 24 hours later the nursing staff noticed that she was confused and generally drowsy. On the following morning she was found in her bed unconscious, with fixed dilated pupils unreactive to light. She had been doubly incontinent. Respiration was irregular, doll's eye movements absent and corneal jerks barely present; the gag reflex was also absent. She responded to painful stimuli by assuming a decorticate posture. Occasionally she would make spontaneous semi-purposeful movements. Reflexes were generally brisk, with the left plantar reflex extensor and the right equivocal. The fundi were normal. Pulse was a regular 60 beats/min, blood pressure was 130/100 mmHg.

Investigations

HAEMATOLOGY & RADIOLOGY
Hb: 14.2 g/dl (14.2 g/100 ml); MCV: 106 fl (106 μm³); MCH: 29 pg (29 $\mu\mu$g); WBC: 17.2 × 10⁹/l (17,200/mm³); Neutrophils: 81%; Lymphocytes: 11%; Platelets: 102 × 10⁹/l (102,000/mm³); CXR: normal cardiac size, lungs normal; Urinanalysis: normal; Electrocardiogram (ECG): Sinus bradycardia, normal QRS complex; U waves present in leads V_1–V_4.

BIOCHEMISTRY
Urea: 1.2 mmol/l (6.7 mg/100 ml); Bilirubin: 24 μmol/l (1.4 mg/100 ml); Serum glutamic oxaloacetic transaminase (SGOT): 172 iu/l; Alkaline phosphatase: 112 iu/l (16.4 KAU/100 ml); Gamma glutamyl transpeptidase: 230 iu/l.

1. List three essential investigations.

2. Give two possible causes for her deterioration.

CASE II

A 54-year-old woman was referred for investigation of weight loss and a pyrexia of unknown origin. She had been well until eight months previously when she first noticed episodes of night sweats and a constant feeling of tiredness. During these sweats, her temperature would rise to 39°C. She was admitted to a local hospital where twelve successive blood cultures, taken during episodes of pyrexia, were all negative.

She began to lose weight and complained of aches over her bones. She could no longer settle into a comfortable position. On some days she would feel perfectly well, on others she would feel lethargic and complain of 'flu-like' symptoms, associated invariably with a swinging pyrexia. Examination at the first hospital had failed to reveal any significant physical signs; however, a peri-cardial effusion was noted on echocardiography, but aspiration of a small quantity of serosanginous fluid had failed to yield a diagnosis. On admission, she was slightly anaemic, with no clubbing or jaundice. Her arm muscles were tender to palpitation and the left elbow joint was slightly swollen. No other physical abnormality was noted.

Investigations

HAEMATOLOGY
Hb: 9.6 g/dl (9.6 g/100 ml); MCV: 86 fl (86 μm³); ESR: 125 mm/h; Blood film: normocytic normochromic.

BIOCHEMISTRY
Bilirubin: 15 μmol/l (0.8 mg/100 ml); SGOT: 35 iu/l; Albumin: 32 g/l (3.2 g/100 ml); Globulin: 36 g/l (3.6 g/100 ml); Serum electrophoresis: increase in gamma globulin and raised α_2 globulins present; Urinary Bence-Jones proteins: negative.

SEROLOGY
Brucella serology: negative; Viral antibody screen: negative.

RADIOLOGY
Chest X-ray, barium meal and follow-through, barium enema, IVP IVP and abdominal CT scan: all normal; Bone scan and skeletal survey: normal; Gallium scan: normal.

SPECIAL INVESTIGATIONS
Bone marrow: a slight excess of plasma cells noted, some immature plasma cells also present; Bone marrow culture for mycobacterium tuberculosis: negative at 6 weeks; Liver biopsy: granulomas present in the portal tracts — features suggesting a reactive hepatitis; Urine microscopy and culture: normal.

1. What is the most likely underlying diagnosis?

2. Suggest two further investigations which might be helpful diagnostically.

CASE III

A 46-year-old man was admitted to hospital for investigation of jaundice and easy bruising. He had been well until two weeks before, when he developed nausea and 'colicky' abdominal pain with episodes of diarrhoea. A pyrexia of 39°C ensued and he began to complain of headaches. On the day of admission, his friend found him confused and complaining of severe muscular pains. In his past medical history he had been well, apart from duodenal ulcers. He had recently reduced his alcohol consumption considerably but still smoked twenty cigarettes daily. He had never held a steady job but recently had accepted casual labour from the local council.

On examination he had a pyrexia of 38.5°C, and was icteric. Urine was dark and contained bile on dipstick testing. Petechiae were noted over the chest and abdomen. A large ecchymosis was noted near the knee joint. Pulse was a regular 120 beats/min and blood pressure was 190/125 mmHg. The heart was clinically enlarged and auscultation revealed features of mild mitral regurgitation with evidence of an early diastolic murmur at the left sternal edge. The liver was slightly tender, but no other abnormalities were present. On neurological examination mild neck stiffness was present, but the fundi were normal. Reflexes were symmetrical, and plantars were bilaterally flexor.

Investigations

HAEMATOLOGY
Hb: 12.4g/dl (12.4g/100ml); MCV: 101fl (101μm³); WBC: 24.0 × 10⁹/l (24,000/mm³); Neutrophils: 86%; Platelets: 105 × 10⁹/l (105,000/mm³); PTTK: 42 (normal range: 25-32 sec); Prothrombin time (PT): 16sec (control 14).

BIOCHEMISTRY
Potassium: 5.3mmol/l (5.3mEq/l); Urea: 23.4mmol/l (212mg/100ml); Chloride: 107mmol/l (107mEq/l); Bicarbonate: 13mmol/l (13mEq/l); Glucose: 6.3mmol/l (113mg/100ml); Bilirubin: 84μmol/l (4.9mg/100ml); SGOT: 128iu/l; Alkaline phosphatase: 174iu/l (22.62KAU/100ml); Albumin: 36g/l (3.6g/100ml); Urinanalysis: protein ++++, red cells ++, bile ++, urobilinogen ++; CSF: protein 0.5g/l (50mg/100ml); glucose: 4.1mmol/l (74mg/100ml), lymphocytic pleocytosis present.

1. List three investigations which might be helpful at this stage.

2. What is the likely diagnosis?

CASE IV

A 47-year-old publican was brought to casualty at 11.00a.m. in a semiconscious state. The only history available was from the patient's sister who said that she had been unable to wake him up that morning.

On examination, the patient's radial pulse was 84 beats/min and regular, and his blood pressure was 150/80mmHg. He responded to painful stimuli, moaned and made some spontaneous movements of his arms and legs. There was no neck stiffness, Kernig's sign was absent, but limb muscle spasticity was present. There were no other abnormalities on physical examination. His temperature was 37.4°C. A lumbar puncture revealed a raised CSF pressure of 200mmH₂O, and there was a free rise and fall in Queckenstedt's test. Several hours later the patient regained full consciousness, but had what appeared to be an expressive dysphasia and mild dysarthria. It subsequently transpired that his speech problem had been long-standing.

On the following day, the patient appeared to have made a complete recovery. The initial electrolyte and haematological results were within normal limits except for an ESR of 82mm/h following admission. The patient was discharged, but over the following four weeks suffered several episodes of weakness affecting his arms and legs, lasting several hours but resolving spontaneously. Six weeks later he was readmitted with a history of acute onset of becoming strange, rigid and immobile. On examination, he again showed generalised muscle spasticity and appeared to be fully conscious but uncommunicative. Within an hour this state ceased and no abnormality could be detected on neurological examination. On chest radiography, consolidation of the basal segments of the left lower lobe and left hilar enlargement were found.

1. List four diagnostically important steps in his management on the second admission.

2. Give a possible diagnosis.

CASE V

A 30-year-old married woman was admitted to hospital as an emergency. Her husband indicated that she had had a drinking problem for nearly two years but, apart from two recent visits to her general practitioner, she had been in good health allowing for her alcohol intake. During the few weeks prior to her last visit she had been drinking more than usual, and this had led to marital disharmony because of the financial and social effects of her drinking. Her 7-year-old son had recently been diagnosed as having diabetes. Following her most recent visit to the GP, the patient had been put on a regular medication but her husband did not know its name or why it was prescribed. Since starting the tablets, she had had occasional episodes of loss of consciousness, vaguely described by her husband as fits. On the morning of admission she was unarousable.

On examination she was unconscious with minimal response to painful stimuli; her breathing was adequate. Reflexes were generally brisk but symmetrical: plantar responses were bilaterally extensor. Intermittent generalised spontaneous twitching was present. She was in sinus rhythm; her pulse was a regular 130 beats/min and her blood pressure was 130/80mmHg. Auscultation of the lungs revealed coarse crackles in the right base. The abdomen was soft, but bowel sounds were noticeably diminished.

Investigations

Hb: 13.4g/dl (13.4g/100ml); ESR: 26mm/h; MCV: 97fl (97μm³); MCH: 29pg (29 $\mu\mu$g); WBC: 11.6 × 10⁹/l (11,600/mm³); Sodium: 136mmol/l (136mEq/l); Potassium: 3.4mmol/l (3.4mEq/l); Urea: 4.6mmol/l (27.8mg/100ml); Bilirubin: 17μmol/l (1mg/100ml); SGOT: 36iu/l; Total protein: 67g/l; Albumin: 34g/l; Urinanalysis: normal.

1. List four essential steps in her immediate management.

2. What is the most likely diagnosis?

Data Interpretations

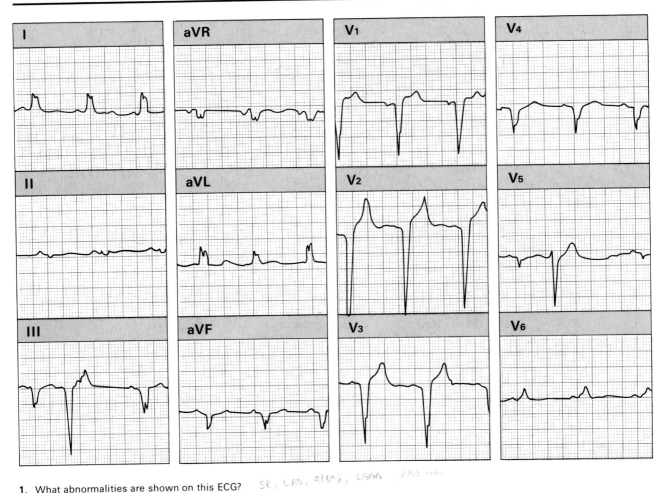

1. What abnormalities are shown on this ECG? 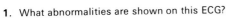 SR, LAD, QRST↓, LBBB ... ?/5/? ...

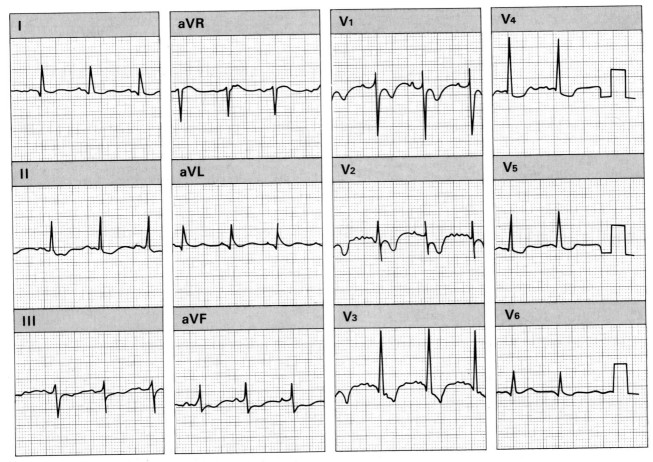

1.8 2. What abnormalities are shown?

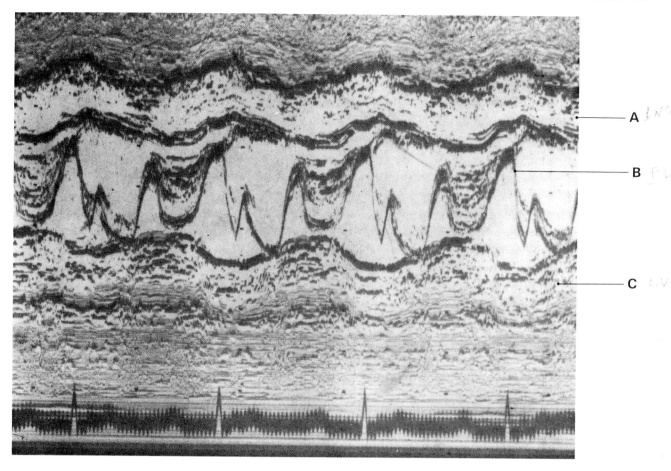

A *LN*

B *PL*

C *L.V*

3. **(a)** Name structures A, B, C in this M mode echocardiogram.
   (b) What is the diagnosis? *LAN / MVP*

4. Give three possible causes for the following biochemistry:
   T4: 212nmol/l (normal range: 58-174nmol/l); THUT: 154 (normal range: 92-118); FTI: 187 (normal range: 58-174); T3: 4.8nmol/l (normal range: 1.23-3.07nmol/l); TSH: 1.5mU/l (normal range: 0.4-6mU/l).

5. A 16-year-old girl being treated for diabetic ketoacidosis has the following biochemistry:
   Sodium: 138mmol/l (138mEq/l); Potassium: 4.8nmol/l (4.8mEq/l); Chloride: 112mmol/l (112mEq/l); Bicarbonate: 14mmol/l (14mEq/l); pH: 7.28; Lactic acid: 3mmol/l; Urine ketones: negative.
   (a) What type of acidosis is present?
   (b) List three conditions in which this type of acidosis may be found.

6. A male, aged 64 years, complains of nausea and vomiting. His investigations were as follows:
   Hb: 7.9g/dl (7.9g/100ml); PCV: 0.3 (30%); MCV: 85fl (85μm³); MCH: 30pg (30μμg); MCHC: 33g/dl (33g/100ml); ESR: 131mm/h, reticulocyte count: 1%; Platelets: 91 × 10⁹/l (91,000/mm³); WBC: 8.1 × 10⁹/l (8,100/mm³); Film: Nucleated red cells present; Rouleaux +++.
   (a) List four helpful investigations.
   (b) Suggest a possible diagnosis.

7. A 16-year-old girl is investigated after a 12-day history of jaundice and persistent lethargy.
   Bilirubin: 94μmol/l (5.5mg/100ml); SGOT: 89iu/l; Alkaline phosphatase: 194iu/l; Urinanalysis: bile and urobilinogen present; Blood film: lymphocytosis, relative neutropenia; Reticulocyte count: 6.3%.
   (a) List two investigations which would be helpful diagnostically.
   (b) What is the most likely diagnosis?

8. A 14-year-old boy being investigated for short stature has the following biochemistry:
   Urea: 6.2mmol/l (38mg/100ml); Sodium: 140mmol/l (140mEq/l); Potassium: 2.8mmol/l (2.8mEq/l); Chloride: 114mmol/l (114mEq/l); Bicarbonate: 14mmol/l (14mEq/l); Alkaline phosphatase: 146iu/l; Albumin: 37g/dl (3.7g/100ml).
   (a) How would you describe this biochemical defect?
   (b) List two investigations which would elucidate the underlying diagnosis.

9. A 6-year-old child was found unconscious with a temperature of 38.2°C. Investigations:
   CSF examination: lymphocytes: 4 × 10⁶/l (4/mm³), proteins: 0.5g/l (50mg/100ml), glucose: 3.3mmol/l (59.4mg/100ml); Urea: 9mmol/l (54mg/100ml); Plasma bicarbonate: 11mmol/l (11mEq/l).
   (a) List two important investigations.
   (b) Suggest a likely diagnosis.

10. A 64-year-old woman is investigated for intractable pruritus. She is noted to have shingles of the L1 and L2 segments.
    Hb: 10.8g/dl (10.8g/100ml); PCV: 0.35 (35%); MCV: 85fl (85μm³); WBC: 27 × 10⁹/l (27,000/mm³); Neutrophils: 28%; Lymphocytes: 64%; Monocytes: 2%; Eosinophils: 1%; Reticulocytes: 3.4%; Platelets: 87 × 10⁹/l (87,000/mm³); Film: spherocytes +++, smudge cells +; Alkaline phosphatase: 94iu/l; Bilirubin: 38μmol/l.
    (a) What is the probable cause of the anaemia?
    (b) What is the most likely underlying diagnosis?

Answers

ANSWERS TO SLIDE INTERPRETATIONS

Key: Ideal answer: ★★★★   Some credit for: ★
Possible answer: ★★   No credit for: 0

1. **(a)** Gingival hyperplasia ★★★★
   (b) Cyclosporin therapy ★★★★
   Phenytoin ★★

2. **(a)** Xanthelasmata ★★★★
   Periorbital purpura ★★★★
   (b) Amyloidosis ★★★★
   Hyperlipidaemia ★★
   Spontaneous purpura, particularly in the head and neck region, is characteristic of amyloidosis. It is caused mainly by capillary fragility due to amyloid infiltration of small vessels. Amyloid infiltration of the kidneys will cause a nephrotic syndrome, which is associated with hyperlipidaemia (hence the xanthelasmata here).

3. Choroidal naevus ★★★★
   Melanoma ★
   Choroidoretinitis 0

4. **(a)** Acute ulcerative colitis ★★★★
   (b) Bacillary dysentery, e.g. Shigella ★★
   Campylobacter enteritis ★★
   Amoebic dysentery ★
   Crohn's disease 0
   Ischaemic colitis 0

5. Paget's disease ★★★★
   Osteomyelitis, syphilis 0

6. Poliomyelitis ★★★★
   Hemiatrophy of limb ★
   Motor neurone disease 0

7. Pericardial disease ★★★★
   Tuberculous pericarditis ★★
   A gross fibrinous epicardial surface with an area of caseation.
   Pericarditis may be the first sign of underlying tuberculous infection.

8. Charcot-Marie-Tooth disease ★★★★
   Refsum's disease ★★★★
   Friedreich's ataxia ★★★★
   Leprosy ★★★★
   Dupuytren's contraction 0
   Ulnar nerve palsy 0

9. **(a)** Hydrocephalus ★★★★
   Calcified lesion in third ventricle ★★★★
   (b) Craniopharyngioma ★★★★
   Ependymoma, pituitary tumour ★★
   Colloid cyst of third ventricle 0

10. Sigmoid volvulus ★★★★
    Caecal volvulus ★
    Volvulus ★
    Sigmoid volvulus occurs typically in old age or in psychiatrically disturbed, mentally retarded or institutionalised people. The mechanism is twisting of the sigmoid loop around its mesenteric axis. It is usually a chronic condition, with intermittent acute attacks. A barium enema should be carried out to confirm the diagnosis.

11. Panphotocoagulation of the eyes ★★★★
    Laser therapy ★★★

12. **(a)** Fixed drug eruption ★★★★
    Drug eruption ★★
    Drug-induced eczema ★
    Allergic rash ★
    (b) Phenolphthalein, Sulphonamides or Penicillin ★★★★

13. Hurler's syndrome ★★★★
    There is flattening of the nasal bridge and acrocephaly. These are the typical features of Hurler's syndrome.

14. **(a)** Swelling of proximal interphalangeal joints ★★★★
    Tophus over knuckle and proximal interphalangeal joint of third toe ★★★★
    (b) Gout ★★★★
    Rheumatoid arthritis with rheumatoid nodule 0

15. Herpes simplex (Herpes genitalis) infection ★★★★
    Syphilitic chancre ★
    Pilonidal sinus 0

16. The Leser–Trélat syndrome ★★★★
    Seborrhoeic warts ★★

17. Retinal artery branch occlusion ★★★★
    Retinal artery occlusion ★★
    Retinal vein thrombosis 0

18. Graves' ophthalmopathy ★★★★
    Thyroid-associated ophthalmopathy ★★★★

19. Extradural haematoma ★★★★
    Subdural haematoma 0
    This is a typical extradural haematoma with convex medial and lateral borders. A subdural, by comparison, has a concave medial border.

20. Coeliac malabsorption pattern ★★★★
    Crohn's disease 0

ANSWERS TO CASE HISTORIES

Case I
1. **(a)** Midbrain bleed ★★★★
   (b) Supratentorial lesion, e.g. subdural haematoma causing brainstem distortion and uncal herniation ★★★★
   Portosystemic encephalopathy ★★

2. Enhanced CT scan ★★★★
   Angiography ★★★★
   Blood glucose level ★★★★
   Potassium level ★★★★
   Radioisotope brain scan ★★
   EEG ★
   Lumbar puncture 0

Case II
1. Giant cell arteritis ★★★★
   Miliary tuberculosis ★★

2. Temporal artery biopsy ★★★★
   Mantoux test ★★
   Pericardial biopsy ★★
   Double-stranded anti-DNA antibody ★

Case III

1. Blood cultures (whole blood should be innoculated into a semi-solid medium, e.g. Fletcher's) ★★★★
   Serology (microscopic haemagglutination test) ★★★★
   Examination of urine for leptospirosis ★★★★
   Echocardiogram ★★

2. Leptospirosis ★★★★
   Meningococcal septicaemia ★★
   Gonococcal septicaemia ★
   Acute bacterial endocarditis ★

Case IV

1. Sputum cytology ★★★★
   Bronchoscopy and biopsy ★★★★
   Blood glucose ★★★★
   CT scan of head ★★★★
   Liver function tests ★★
   CSF bacteriology, protein and sugar estimation ★★
   WR (syphilis serology) ★★
   Ethanol level ★★

2. Paraneoplastic syndrome (with encephalopathy), secondary
      to bronchial carcinoma ★★★★
   Bronchial carcinoma ★★
   Recurrent transient ischaemic attacks ★★
   Hypoglycaemic coma ★
   Portosystemic encephalopathy ★
   Disseminated sclerosis 0
   Viral encephalitis 0

Case V

1. Ensure airway patency ★★★★
   Intravenous line ★★★★
   Cardiac monitor ★★★★
   Insert nasogastric tube ★★★★
   Chest radiograph ★★★★
   Metronidazole and ampicillin therapy for possible
      aspiration ★★★★
   Gastric lavage after insertion of endotracheal tube ★★

2. Tricyclic antidepressant overdose ★★★★

ANSWERS TO DATA INTERPRETATIONS

1. Left bundle branch block ★★★★
   Left axis deviation ★★★★
   Ventricular premature beat ★★★★

2. Anterolateral subendocardial ischaemic changes ★★★★
   Inferior subendocardial changes ★★★★

3. (a) A = Interventricular septum ★★★★
      B = Anterior leaflet of mitral valve ★★★★
      C = Posterior wall of left ventricle ★★★★
   (b) Left atrial myxoma ★★★★
   There is a characteristic dense mass of echos behind the ALMV,
   characteristically preceded by an echo-free space at the mitral
   valve of the onset of diastole, reflecting the time required for the
   atrial myxoma to prolapse through the mitral valve orifice.

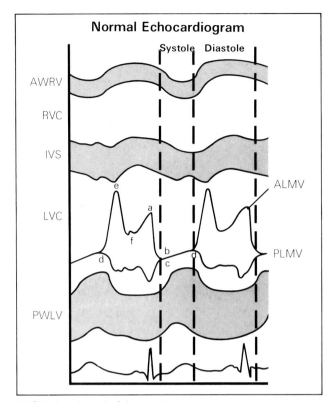

AWRV: Anterior wall of right ventricle
RVC: Right ventricular cavity
IVS: Interventricular septum
LVC: Left ventricular cavity
PWLV: Posterior wall of left ventricle
ALMV: Anterior leaflet of mitral valve
PLMV: Posterior leaflet of mitral valve

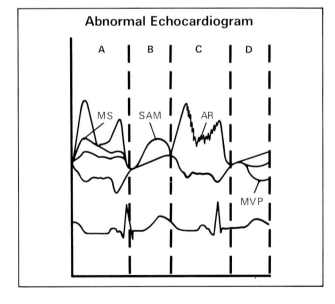

A = Mitral Stenosis (MS): Both anterior and posterior leaflets move
      anteriorly during diastole, and the EF slope is greatly diminished.
B = 'HOCM': During systole, there is systolic anterior movement
      (SAM) of the anterior leaflet of the mitral valve, sometimes to the
      point of touching the interventricular septum.
C = Aortic Regurgitation (AR): There is a characteristic fluttering of the
      anterior mitral valve leaflet during diastole caused by the
      impinging aortic regurgitated jet (responsible for the Austin-Flint
      murmur).
D = Mitral Valve Prolapse (MVP): During late systole, the leaflets move
      posteriorly, especially the posterior leaflet of the mitral valve.

4. Hereditary TBG excess ★★★
   Contraceptive pill ★★★★
   Phenothiazines ★★★★
   Clofibrate therapy ★★★★
   Pregnancy ★★★★
   Thyrotoxicosis 0

5. (a) Hyperchloraemic acidosis ★★★★
   (b) Use of a carbonic anhydrase inhibitor ★★★★
      Renal tubular acidosis ★★★★
      Uretero-sigmoidostomy ★★★★

6. (a) Skeletal survey ★★★★
      Serum calcium ★★★★
      Urinary Bence-Jones protein ★★★★
      Serum electrophoresis ★★★★
      Bone marrow aspirate ★★★★
   (b) Myeloma ★★★★
      Miliary TB ★★
      Carcinomatosis ★★

7. (a) Paul-Bunnell test ★★★★
      EBV titres ★★★★
      Hepatitis A IgM antibody ★★
      HBs Ag ★
   (b) Hepatitis probably secondary to infectious
      monocucleosis ★★★★
      Viral hepatitis ★

8. (a) Hyperchloraemic acidosis ★★★★
   (b) Urinary amino acids, phosphate, glucose,
      bicarbonate ★★★★
      Plain radiograph of kidneys ★★★★
      Urinary acidification test ★★★★
   The most likely diagnosis here is renal tubular acidosis.

9. (a) Salicylate levels in blood ★★★★
      Blood gases ★★★★
      Cardiac monitor ★★★★
      Plasma electrolytes ★★★★
      Blood glucose ★★
      Chest X-ray ★
   (b) Salicylate intoxication ★★★★

10. (a) Autoimmune haemolytic anaemia ★★★★
      Aplastic anaemia 0
   (b) Chronic lymphocytic leukaemia (CLL) ★★★★
      Viral lymphocytosis 0
   CLL accounts for 25% of leukaemias seen in clinical practice.
   Superficial lymphadenopathy, hepatosplenomegaly, thrombocytopenia and anaemia are common. Bone marrow aspiration
   shows lymphocytic replacement of normal marrow elements,
   with (usually 'B') lymphocytes comprising 25–95% of all cells.
   Reduced concentrations of serum immunoglobulins are found in
   most patients, particularly with advanced disease. The
   lymphocytes themselves have surface-bound immunoglobulins of
   IgM and IgD type, and membrane receptors for the Fc fragment
   of IgG and for C3. Haemolysis is usually caused by 'warm'
   autoantibody Coombs' positive haemolytic anaemia.

Paper 2

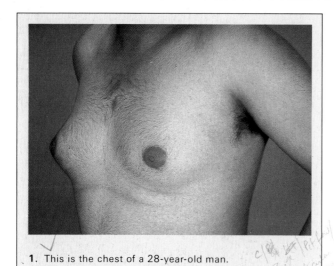

1. This is the chest of a 28-year-old man.
    List three possible causes for this physical sign.

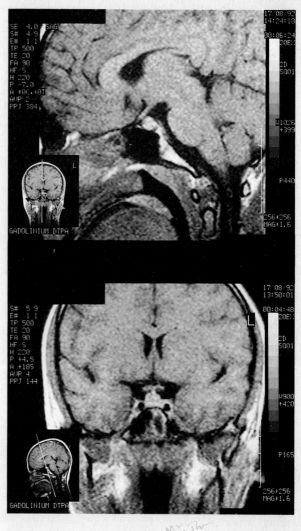

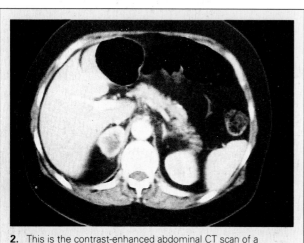

2. This is the contrast-enhanced abdominal CT scan of a
    patient who presented with acute left ventricular failure.
    (a) What is the abnormality?
    (b) What is the most likely diagnosis?

3. **(a)** What is the investigation?
    (b) What abnormality is shown?

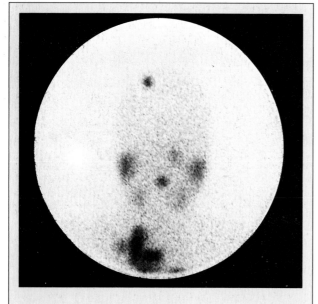

4. What are the two obvious abnormalities on this child's
    chest radiograph?

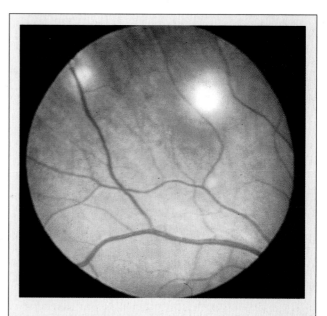

5. This is the fundus of a 35-year-old Indian woman with
    drowsiness and mild neck stiffness.
    Suggest a likely cause for the abnormality shown.

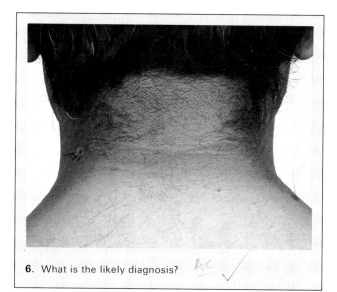

6. What is the likely diagnosis?

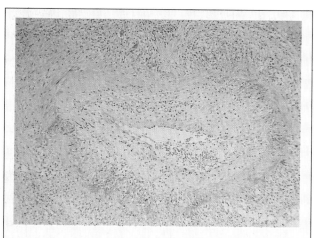

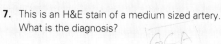

7. This is an H&E stain of a medium sized artery. What is the diagnosis?

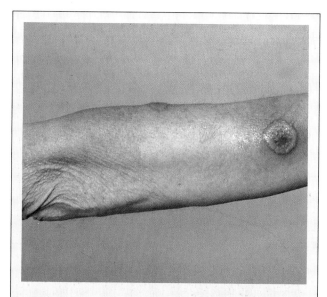

8. This lesion had developed five days before, as an extremely tender cluster of subcutaneous nodules which seemed to coalesce and then ulcerate. What is the most likely diagnosis?

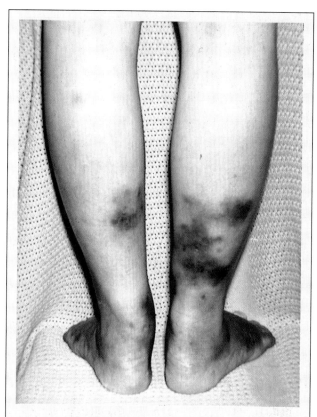

9. These are the legs of a 55-year-old woman being treated for a pulmonary condition. What is the likely diagnosis?

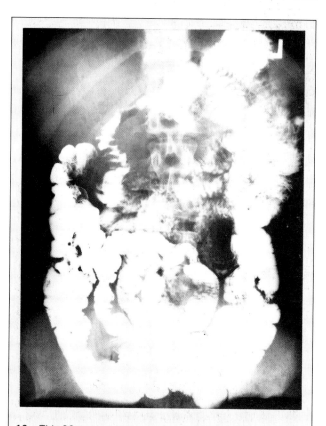

10. This 20-year-old Asian male complained of abdominal pain.
    (a) What study is shown?
    (b) What is the diagnosis?

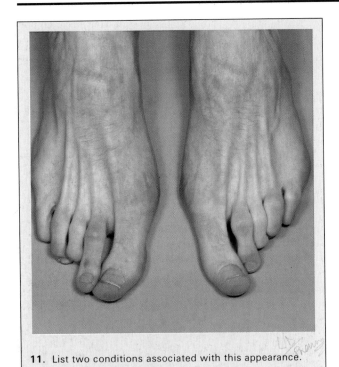

11. List two conditions associated with this appearance.

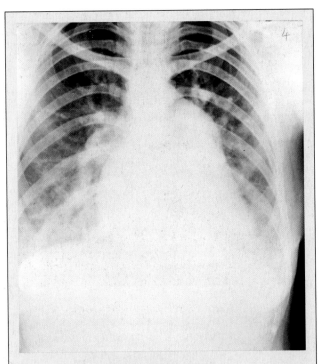

12. This is the chest radiograph of a middle-aged woman with recent onset of right heart failure.
What is the most likely cause of this appearance?

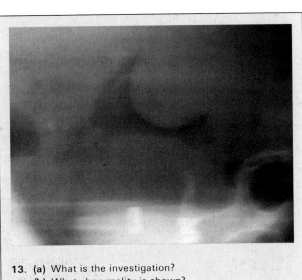

13. (a) What is the investigation?
    (b) What abnormality is shown?

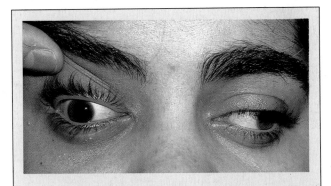

14. This patient is attempting to look to the left.
    (a) What is the most probable diagnosis?
    (b) List two possible causes.

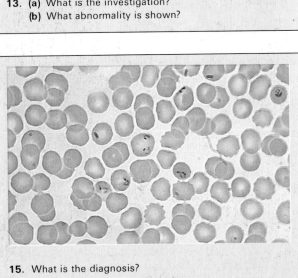

15. What is the diagnosis?

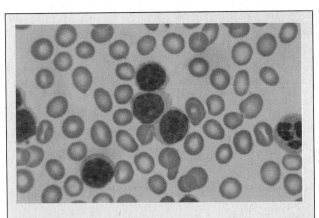

16. This is the blood film of a 51-year-old man with fatigue. A few lymph nodes were palpable in the axillae.
What is the likely diagnosis?

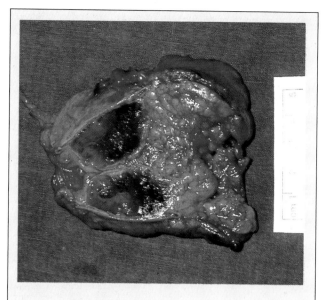

17. This is the left adrenal gland of a patient who died of acute pulmonary oedema.
What is the diagnosis?

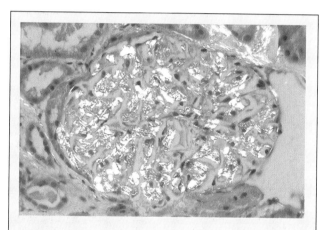

18. This is a renal biopsy specimen from a patient with heavy proteinuria, viewed under polarised light.
What abnormality is shown?

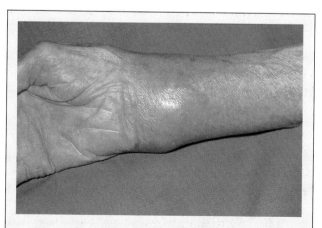

19. This 84-year-old lady developed an acute swollen wrist overnight. The joint aspirate was sterile.
What is the most likely diagnosis?

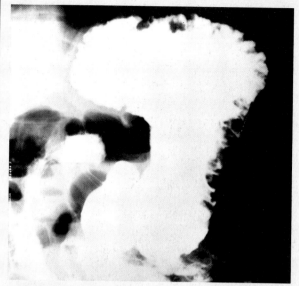

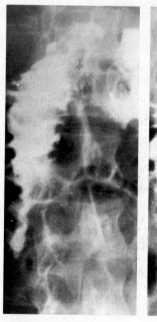 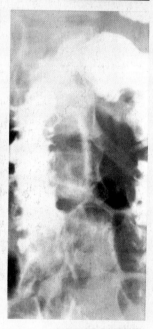

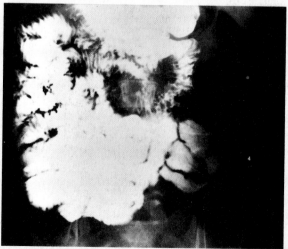

20. This barium study was carried out in a 40-year-old woman with a long history of recurrent peptic ulceration, and recent onset of watery diarrhoea.
(a) What abnormality is present?
(b) Suggest the most likely diagnosis.

CASE I

A 31-year-old school teacher was admitted for investigation of dizzy spells and several episodes of loss of consciousness. According to his wife, he had been well until six months before, when one morning she found it difficult to wake him up. The GP was called in, but by the time he arrived the patient was awake and complaining of a headache. No obvious cause could be found for this episode.Two weeks later, after drinking a pint of beer, he became unusually drowsy – this lasted for about ten minutes. Following this, his wife remarked that he became talkative and was speaking nonsense for a further ten minutes, during which time he was sweating profusely. Two weeks before admission he had two epileptiform seizures at a party. Since then, he had been complaining of feeling unsteady on his feet. There was no past medical history of note, but on questioning it appeared that over the previous two months he had gained one stone in weight.

On examination, he was a well-looking man and very terse in his replies. Pulse was 70/min regular, blood pressure 130/90mmHg. Examination of the cardiovascular system, including peripheral pulses, was normal. Lungs were clear, and abdominal examination was unremarkable. His reflexes were brisk but tone was normal, and plantar reflexes were flexor.

Investigations

HAEMATOLOGY
Hb: 15.1g/dl (15.1g/100ml); MCV: 84fl (84μm^3); WBC: 6×10^9/l (6,000/mm^3); Normal differential count; ESR: 12mm/h; Platelets: 560×10^9 (560,000/mm^3).

BIOCHEMISTRY
Urea: 3.6mmol/l (21.8mg/100ml); Glucose: 4.2mmol/l (84mg/dl); Creatinine: 0.08μmol/l (0.8mg/100ml); Sodium: 138mmol/l (138mEq/l); Potassium: 3.3mmol/l (3.3mEq/l); Bicarbonate: 24mmol/l (24mEq/l); Chloride: 97mmol/l (97mEq/l); Liver function tests: normal; Calcium: 2.78mmol/l (10.9mg/100ml); Phosphate: 0.64mmol/l (0.64mEq/l); Alkaline phosphatase: 50iu/l (6.5 KAU/100ml); Albumin: 46g/l (4.6g/100ml); Urinanalysis: normal.

RADIOLOGY
CXR: heart size normal, lungs clear; ECG: normal QRS axis, no ST segment abnormalities.

1. List four investigations which would assist in the management of this patient.

2. List two possible diagnoses.

CASE II

A 55-year-old woman was admitted to hospital for investigation of episodic transient cerebral ischaemic attacks. She had been hypertensive for seven years, and two years prior to admission she had been noted by her GP to have mild carotid bruits. Eight weeks, and again four days, before admission she had developed sudden onset of an expressive dysphasia and mild right hemiparesis. On the second occasion, her blood pressure was found to be 270/140mmHg and the patient was referred for urgent admission.

On examination, her hypertension was confirmed and she was noted to have mild pyramidal weakness on the right side with some nominal dysphasia and evidence of a right homonymous hemianopia. Prominent carotid bruits were noted particularly on the left side, and the heart was found to be slightly enlarged with a hyperdynamic apex. Initial investigations showed normal full blood count and electrolytes, and a normal liver function test. Over the course of three days her neurological disability recovered fully, and her blood pressure was brought under control with labetalol and bethanidine. In view of her relatively young age, an angiographic study of her neck vessels was carried out via a right femoral artery puncture. This showed severe atherosclerotic changes at the left carotid bifurcation, and some atherosclerotic disease of the carotid syphon. The left vertebral artery was irregular. The patient once again became dysphasic with a recurrence of the right-sided weakness immediately following the procedure. Accordingly, she was heparinised and then put on oral anticoagulants. Within two days of the procedure her neurological status once again improved, but she was noted to have become oliguric, with biochemical evidence of deteriorating renal function.

Investigations

Hb: 12.3g/dl (12.3g/100ml); MCV: 92fl (92μm^3); WBC: 10.6×10^9/l (10,600/mm^3); Normal differential count; Sodium: 137mmol/l (137mEq/l); Potassium: 5.2mmol/l (5.2mEq/l); Bicarbonate: 13mmol/l (13mEq/l); Chloride: 107mmol/l (107mEq/l); Urea: 28.6mmol/l (174mg/100ml); Creatinine: 450μmol/l (5.08mg/100ml); (On admission: Urea: 10.2mmol/l, Creatinine: 216μmol/l); Prothrombin time: 18 sec (control 13 sec); Cardiac enzymes: normal; ECG: evidence of LVH and strain; CXR: prominent left ventricle; Urinanalysis: protein +++, red cells ++.

1. List three measures which are indicated in the patient's immediate management.

2. Give two possible reasons for her deteriorating renal function.

CASE III

A 65-year-old Jamaican first presented to his GP in 1976, complaining of a generalised pruritic eruption. This was treated with betnovate cream and improved after two weeks. He was then quite well until 1981, when he was referred to the outpatients department for investigation of unexplained weight loss and epigastric discomfort. Investigations at that time revealed a normal barium meal and follow-through. An ultrasound of the pancreas was normal. His weight loss was ascribed to the onset of diabetes, which was subsequently treated with glibenclamide. In March 1985, he was admitted from the accident and emergency department complaining of feeling generally ill, with a constant pain in his stomach and a three-month history of intermittent, non-bloody diarrhoea. He reported episodes of an itchy eruption involving his back, but this would resolve within a week. There had been a 10kg weight loss.

On examination, the patient appeared thin and unwell. There was generalised abdominal tenderness. His weight was 58kg, and temperature 37.2°C.

Investigations

HAEMATOLOGY

Hb: 13.4g/dl (13.4g/100ml); MCV: 82fl (82μm^3); WBC: 9 × 10^9/l (9,000/mm^3); Neutrophils: 60%; Lymphocytes: 20%; Eosinophils: 16%; Platelets: 285 × 10^9/l (285,000/mm^3); ESR: 55mm/h.

BIOCHEMISTRY

Urea: 6.4mmol/l (39mg/100ml); Sodium: 140mmol/l (140mEq/l); Potassium: 3.8mmol/l (3.8mEq/l); Bicarbonate: 23mmol/l (23mEq/l); Chloride: 98mmol/l (98mEq/l); Bilirubin: 16μmol/l (0.97mg/100ml); Alkaline phosphatase: 68iu/l (9 KAU/100ml); Albumin: 23g/l (2.3g/100ml); Calcium: 1.86mmol/l (7.29mg/100ml); Serum glutamic oxaloacetic transaminase (SGOT): 50iu/l; Red cell folate: 180μg/l; Urinanalysis: normal.

RADIOLOGY & SPECIAL INVESTIGATIONS

CXR: normal; Barium enema: irregular appearance of mucosa suggestive of inflammatory bowel disease; Colonoscopic study: mucosa very inflamed; Biopsy: crypt abscesses ++; Inflammatory change in the submucosa ++.

1. List two investigations which are essential in the management of this patient.

2. Suggest the most likely diagnosis.

CASE IV

A 25-year-old man was admitted for investigation for weakness in his legs. He had been well until six months before, when he first noted jerky movements in his right leg and progressive weakness which was apparent when he climbed stairs. Over the last two months he had become unaware of pain sensations in his right leg, with no other disturbance involving the arms, the cranial nerves or sphincters. The patient had a complex medical history, and had been deaf in the left ear since birth. He had had surgery to his hips between the ages of five and six, and a closure of an atrial septal defect at the age of eight. In his family history it appeared that both his mother and brother had clubbed feet, and his mother had had surgical repair of a cardiac lesion. The patient drank fifteen pints of beer each day and was a heavy smoker.

On examination, he was a well-looking man with abnormal teeth and a mild thoracic scoliosis. Pulse 70/min regular, blood pressure 120/80mmHg. Examination of the heart and lungs was normal, as was abdominal examination. The optic discs looked a little pale, and there was an absent gag reflex. His legs were spastic, and there was bilateral pyramidal weakness worse on the right than on the left. His gait looked spastic, and he was hyperflexic with bilateral extensor plantar responses. There was patchy loss of sensation to pinprick extending from the feet as far as below the nipple line bilaterally, with some preservation of sensation around the buttocks.

Investigations

HAEMATOLOGY

Hb: 18.3g/dl (18.3g/100ml); PCV: 0.54 (54%); MCV: 87fl (87μm^3); WBC: 6.8 × 10^9/l (6,800/mm^3); Normal differential count; ESR: 1mm/h; Platelets: 225 × 10^9/l (225,000/mm^3).

BIOCHEMISTRY & SPECIAL INVESTIGATIONS

Urea and electrolytes: normal; Liver function tests: normal; Blood glucose: 5.6mmol/l (98mg/100ml); Calcium: 2.46mmol/l (9.6 mg/100ml); Phosphate: 0.64mmol/l (0.64mEq/l); Red cell folate: 450μg/l; Karyotype: XY; CXR: scoliosis in the mid thoracic region noted; Heart size: normal; Lung fields: clear; Cervical spine X-ray: AP view normal, but on lateral view there seems to be increase in the posterior diameter of the cervical spine from C1 to C3.

1. List three investigations which would be diagnostically useful.

2. Suggest two possible diagnoses.

CASE V

A 34-year-old farmer was investigated for weakness and pain in his shoulder. He had suffered from heavy flu two weeks before, and over the last two days had developed pain around the left shoulder; this became increasingly severe over a 24-hour period. Later on the pain subsided, but the patient noticed progressive weakness of his shoulder girdle musculature more marked on the left. Over the ensuing days, the weakness in the left arm spread to involve the distal musculature.

On examination, he was a well-looking man and apyrexial. Examination of his upper limbs showed severe weakness of the left supra- and infraspinatus muscles with weakness of the deltoid, biceps, brachioradialis and triceps being obvious on the left. On the right, there was marked weakness of the supra- and infraspinatus and deltoid muscles, and mild weakness of the biceps and brachioradialis muscle. All deep tendon reflexes in the upper limbs were absent except for the right triceps. Cranial nerve examination was unremarkable, and the remainder of the neurological examination was normal.

Investigations

Hb: 15.2g/dl (15.2 g/100ml); WBC: 6.4 × 10^9/l (6,000/mm^3); ESR: 33mm/h; Urea and electrolytes: normal; Liver function tests: normal; CXR: normal; Urinanalysis: normal.

What is the most likely diagnosis?

Data Interpretations

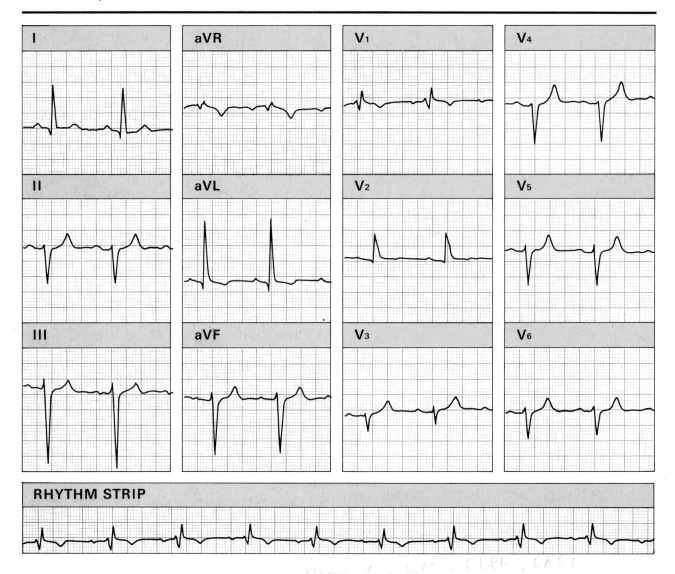

I	aVR	V₁	V₄
II	aVL	V₂	V₅
III	aVF	V₃	V₆

RHYTHM STRIP

1. List three abnormalities on this ECG.

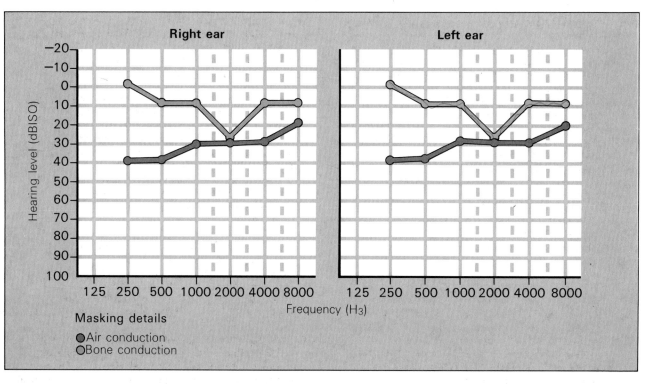

2. What is the most likely cause of this audiometric appearance?

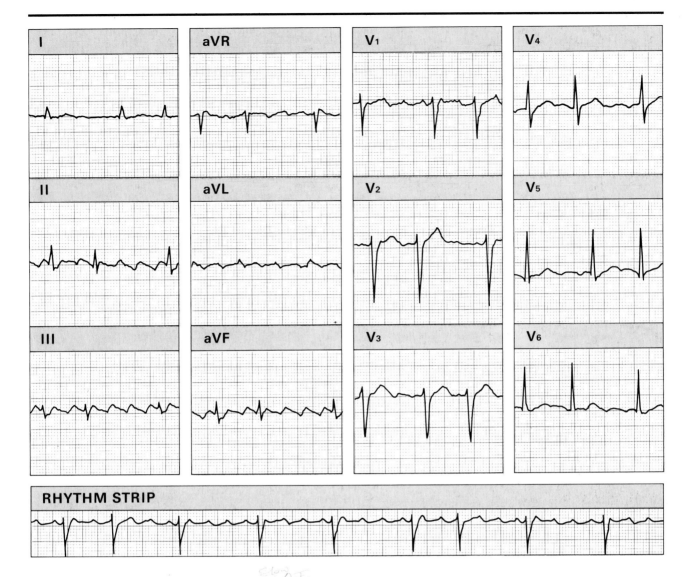

I	aVR	V₁	V₄

II	aVL	V₂	V₅

III	aVF	V₃	V₆

RHYTHM STRIP

3. What is the electrocardiographic diagnosis?

4. A 34-year old woman gave a three day history of lower abdominal pain and dysuria. She was admitted with a tense swollen right knee, which was aspirated.
Turbid fluid; Cytology: neutrophils ++++; No crystals found; Glucose content: 1.6mmol/l; Aerobic culture: negative; Peripheral WBC: 16.4×10^9/l (16,400/mm³).
(a) List three essential investigations.
(b) Suggest two possible diagnoses.

5. A 23-year-old woman gives a short history of malaise and fever. On examination, lymphadenopathy is found.
Hb: 14.2g/dl (14.2g/100ml); WBC: 8.6×10^9/l (8,600/mm³); (25% atypical). A heterophil antibody test is carried out: no absorption: +; after absorption on ox red cells: +; after absorption on guinea pig kidney: −.
(+ = agglutination with sheep red cells; − = no agglutination with sheep red cells).
(a) What inferences can be drawn from these results?
(b) Suggest a possible diagnosis.

6. A 34-year-old man is admitted to hospital with a short history of recurrent transient ischaemic attacks. He has noticed purpurae on his body, and BP is 180/110mmHg.
Hb: 7.8g/dl (7.8g/100ml); WBC: 11.4×10^9/l (11,400/mm³); Platelets: 52×10^9/l (52,000/mm³); Reticulocytes: 3.7%; Urea: 37.8mmol/l (229mg/100ml); Sodium: 127mmol/l (127 mEq/l); Potassium: 6.2mmol/l (6.2mEq/l); Blood film: microspherocytes ++, red cell fragments ++.
Give two possible diagnoses.

7. A 24-year-old woman complained of flitting arthralgia.
Hb: 12.4g/dl (12.4g/100ml); ESR: 80mm/h; RA latex test: negative; VDRL: positive.
(a) List three essential investigations.
(b) Give a possible diagnosis.

8. A 63-year-old man gives a progressive history of nausea, weakness and lethargy. On examination, a sallow complexion is noted, and the conjunctivae are pale.
Hb: 7.2g/dl (7.2g/100ml); Blood film: normocytic normochromic anaemia; Urea: 48.8 mmol/l (254mg/100ml); Sodium: 140mmol/l (140mEq/l); Potassium: 5.6mmol/l (5.6mEq/l); Bicarbonate: 24mmol/l (24mEq/l); Chloride: 96mmol/l (96mEq/l); $PaCO_2$: 5.2kPa (37mmHg); pH: 7.4.
(a) What acid-base disturbance is shown?
(b) Suggest a possible cause.

9. A man with chronic liver failure is admitted following a severe bout of gastroenteritis.
Sodium: 134mmol/l (134mEq/l); Potassium: 3.6mmol/l (3.6mEq/l); Bicarbonate: 10mmol/l (10mEq/l); Chloride: 112mmol/l (112mEq/l); $PaCO_2$: 2.2kPa (17mmHg); pH: 7.38.
Categorise the biochemical/physiological abnormalities present.

10 A 65-year-old man is investigated following a seizure.
Sodium: 112mmol/l (112mEq/l; Potassium: 3.9mmol/l (3.9mEq/l); Plasma osmolality: 238mOsm/kg; Urinary osmolality: 560mOsm/kg. **(a)** What abnormality is shown?
(b) Suggest two possible causes.

Answers

ANSWERS TO SLIDE INTERPRETATIONS

1. Leydig (oestrogen secreting) tumour of testis ★★★★
    Drug therapy: Spironolactone ★★★★
    Oestrogens ★★★★
    Digoxin ★★
    Thyrotoxicosis ★★★★
    Chronic liver disease ★★
    Prolactinoma 0
    Gynaecomastia may occasionally be seen in thyrotoxicosis. It may be aetiologically related to the rise in SHBG which, by binding testosterone, will reduce free circulating testosterone and thus increase the free E_2/testosterone ratio.

2. (a) Right adrenal phaeochromocytoma ★★★★
        Right adrenal tumour ★★
    (b) Phaeochromocytoma/catecholamine-secreting tumour ★★★★
        Conn's adenoma ★
    These are the typical appearances of adrenal phaeochromocytoma.

3. (a) Gallium-enhanced MRI scan ★★★★
        CT scan 0
    (b) Enlarged pituitary gland ★★★★
        Pituitary tumour ★★★★

4. Metastatic paraganglioma ★★★★
    The radionuclide used was ^{123}I-MIGB, which is a chromaffin-seeking radionuclide. In this instance, it has been taken up by some thoracic paragangliomas, and there is a metastatic lesion in the skull. The symmetrical uptake in the head represents salivary gland uptake.

5. Choroidal tubercle ★★★★
    Cytoid bodies associated with systemic lupus erythematosus ★★
    Retinal cytomegalovirus infection ★★
    Choroiditis ★★
    Sarcoidosis ★★
    The ocular manifestations of tuberculosis include:
    Phlyctenular keratoconjunctivitis, which is an allergic external ocular inflammation observed in children at the time of primary infection, and characterised by small blisters (phlyctenules) at the junction of the conjunctiva and cornea; .
    Chloroidal tubercles, as shown here, indicative of disseminated tuberculosis. They produce no symptoms and are difficult to distinguish from other retinal exudates.

6. Acanthosis nigricans ★★★★
    Ethnic pigmentation ★
    Photosensitive lichenoid reaction ★
    There is a brown-black velvety creased skin change in the nuchal fold, blending into normal adjacent skin. Acanthosis nigricans can affect body folds, and favours flexural surfaces. Histologically there is epidermal thickening and folding over a hypertrophic papillary layer.
    Acanthosis nigricans may be associated with:
    Visceral malignancy – usually adenocarcinoma: stomach (70%), colon, oesophagus;
    Insulin-resistant diabetes mellitus;
    Acromegaly; Prader-Willi syndrome;
    Rarely following diethylstilboestrol, corticosteroids or nicotinic acid.

7. Giant cell arteritis ★★★★
    Polyarteritis nodosa 0
    The walls of involved vessels exhibit features more like granulomatous than acute neutrophilic infiltration. Multinuclear giant cells are characteristic, and tend to be arranged circumferentially, apparently in relation to degenerate fragments of the internal elastic lamina.

8. Pyoderma gangrenosum ★★★★
    Ecthyma ★★
    Polyarteritis nodosa ★
    Pyoderma gangrenosum may occur with rheumatoid arthritis, inflammatory bowel disease, Wegener's granulomatosis, lymphoma and plasma cell dyscrasia.
    Pyoderma grangrenosum is a destructive, necrotising non-infective ulceration of the skin which presents as a furuncle-like nodule, pustule or haemorrhagic bulla. The histological changes are not pathognomonic and show features of a large sterile abscess formation in which venous and capillary thrombosis, haemorrhage, necrosis and massive cell infiltration are present.

9. Erythema induratum (Bazin's disease) ★★★★
    Erythema nodosum 0
    This is a form of nodular tuberculid, a form of cutaneous vasculitis found in association with tuberculous infection. Erythema induratum is found exclusively in women. Lumpy indurated lesions, very dark in colour, develop around the ankles and legs. These may break down into ragged-edged, shallow ulcers with a notably indolent course. Although evidence of tuberculosis elsewhere in the body is often lacking, the patients show a high degree of tuberculin sensitivity and the lesions respond to treatment with anti-tuberculous drugs.

10. (a) Barium follow-through ★★★★
        Barium meal 0
    (b) Ascaris infection ★★★★
    This is common in children from Asia, Africa and Central America. Up to 10% may have associated biliary ascariasis which may give rise to obstructive jaundice/cholangitis or liver abscesses. Worms may calcify or show as lucent filling defects in contrast studies (as shown).

11. Congenital contractural arachnodactyly ★★★★
    Marfan's syndrome ★★★★
    Klinefelter's syndrome ★★
    Hypogonadism ★★
    Sipple's syndrome ★★
    Sickle cell anaemia ★★
    Homocystinuria ★★
    All the above conditions may be associated with arachnodactyly.

12. Atrial septal defect (ASD) ★★★★
    Left to right shunt ★★
    Pulmonary embolus 0
    There is cardiomegaly, pulmonary plethora and a small aortic knuckle. The pulmonary trunk is prominent. These appearances are highly suggestive of an ASD.

13. (a) Air encephalogram ★★★★
    (b) Mass within third ventricle ★★★★
        Colloid cyst of third ventricle ★★★★
        Ependymoma ★★
        Craniopharyngioma ★
    This was a colloid cyst of the third ventricle. These can produce increased pressure by occluding the foramina of Monro. Colloid cysts are usually mobile, and obstruction may be intermittent with sudden episodes of headache of the utmost severity. Hydrocephalus and drop attacks may occur.

14. (a) Complete right-sided third nerve palsy ★★★★
        Third nerve palsy ★★
    (b) Surgical section of third nerve ★★★★
        Posterior communicating artery aneurysm ★★★★
        Trauma ★★★★
        Basal meningitis (e.g. tuberculosis, sarcoidosis) ★★★★
        Meningovascular syphilis ★★★★
        Aneurysmal dilatation of intracavernous portion of carotid artery ★★★★

Mononeuritis multiplex, e.g.:
Diabetes mellitus ★★
Rheumatoid arthritis ★★
Polyarteritis nodosa ★★

15. Falciparum malaria ★★★★
Malaria ★★
The blood film shows severe parasitaemia. The characteristic findings on thin film examination of falciparum malaria include:
Predominance of ring forms, often multiple within a single red cell;
Rings with thread-like cytoplasm, double nuclei;
Gametocytes which are banana-shaped.

16. Chronic lymphatic leukaemia ★★★★
Lymphocytosis ★★
Acute lymphoblastic leukaemia 0
Chronic granulocytic leukaemia 0
The characteristic feature here is the raised lymphocyte count. The average count in CLL is around 100×10^9/l. In this condition, the lymphocytes are very readily damaged in the preparation of smears, and so-called smudge (or basket) cells are frequently seen. The majority of cases involve B lymphocytes.

17. Phaeochromocytoma ★★★★
Paraganglioma ★
Conn's adenoma 0
Phaeochromocytomas are usually well circumscribed, rounded masses, whose size may vary greatly (up to 2,274g in one series). The cut surface is usually greyish brown ('phaeo' means grey or dun-coloured), usually with cystic and haemorrhagic areas.

18. Renal amyloidosis ★★★★
Membranous glomerulopathy 0
The amyloid substance characteristically stains pink-red with Congo-Red, and exhibits a pale green birefringence under polarised light. Primary and secondary forms of amyloid are not distinguishable by light microscopy. Thioflavin stains also cause amyloid deposits to fluoresce under ultraviolet light. By microscopy, deposits of amyloid may be seen in the mesangium, capillary, arteriolar walls, tubules and collecting ducts.

19. Pseudogout or pyrophosphate arthropathy/synovitis ★★★★
Acute septic arthritis ★
Crystal synovitis ★
Acute pyrophosphate synovitis may present with an acute systemic reaction with malaise, fever, high ESR, and sometimes a leucocytosis. It may be distinguished from acute septic arthritis by the presence of radiological chondrocalcinosis, and birefringent crystals in the synovial fluid.

20. (a) Thickening of gastric and duodenal folds ★★★★
Peptic ulcer 0
(b) Zollinger Ellison syndrome (with pancreatic disease) ★★★★
Lymphoma of stomach and small bowel ★★
Other causes of rugal hypertrophy include:
Ménétrièr's disease;
Crohn's disease.

ANSWERS TO CASE HISTORIES

Case I

1. Fasting blood glucose and insulin/C peptide ★★★★
72 hour fast with repeated glucose, insulin, C peptide estimations ★★★★
Pancreatic CT scan ★★★★
Pancreatic polypeptide estimation ★★★★

24 hour urinary calcium excretion ★★★★
Parathyroid hormone estimation (PTH) ★★★★
Hydrocortisone suppression test ★★★★
Insulin tolerance test with measurement of insulin and C peptide ★★
Pancreatic ultrasonic scan ★★
Urinary vanillyl mandelic acid (VMA) and metanephrine estimation ★★
Skull X-ray ★★
CT scan of neck ★★
EEG ★★
CT scan of head ★

2. Insulinoma ★★★★
Primary hyperparathyroidism ★★★★
Phaeochromocytoma ★
Transient ischaemic attacks ★
Temporal lobe epilepsy ★
Multiple endocrine neoplasia (Type I) is the most likely underlying diagnosis. This is the association of pancreatic, pituitary and parathyroid neoplasms. The pancreatic tumours can secrete insulin, gastrin, glucagon, somatostatin, GHRH, vasoactive intestinal peptide, and pancreatic polypeptide alone, or in combination. The parathyroid lesions are of the hyperplastic variety, and recently a circulating parathyroid growth and mitogenic factor has been isolated in the plasma of affected patients.

Case II

1. Initiate fluid balance chart ★★★★
Daily fluid restriction to 500ml and volume of urine output ★★★★
Salt restriction ★★★★
Radioisotope renogram ★★★★
High dose IV Frusemide administration ★★★★
Daily weighing ★★
Urine/plasma osmolality ratio determination ★★
Urine/plasma creatinine ratio determination ★★
Urinary sodium estimation ★★
Blood cultures ★★

2. Dissection of descending aorta, causing occlusion of renal arteries ★★★★
Hypotensive episode during arteriography ★★★★
Renal artery embolus ★★
Excessive hypotensive therapy ★★
Anticoagulant-induced renal dysfunction, e.g. interstitial nephropathy with Phenindione 0
There was clearly preexisting renal impairment, probably secondary to hypertensive disease. Renal artery occlusion would have to be bilateral to produce acute renal failure.

Case III

1. Fresh stool microscopy for larvae ★★★★
Strongyloides complement fixation test ★★★★
Duodenal aspirate for larvae ★★★★
Jejunal biopsy for larvae ★★★★
Beal's string test ★★★★
Examination of sputum for larvae ★★

2. Strongyloidiasis ★★★★
Inflammatory bowel disease ★★
Ulcerative colitis ★★
Amoebiasis ★★
The most common gastrointestinal symptom of strongyloidiasis is epigastric pain (often to the right of the midline), constant, and of a dull aching character mimicking a peptic ulcer. Tenderness may also be present. In heavy infection, diarrhoea is common and may be secondary to malabsorption. Large bowel involvement may resemble ulcerative colitis. The diagnosis suggested by the eosinophilia is made by finding the larvae of *Strongyloides stercoralis* in the stool, preferably by using a concentration

Answers

technique. Multi-stool specimens must be examined, as the excretion of larvae may be intermittent. Treatment is with thiabendazole 25mg/kg twice daily for three days.

Case IV

1. Myelography of upper cervical and dorsal regions ★★★★
   CSF examination for malignant cells, oligoclonal bands ★★★★
   Magnetic resonance imaging of cervical spine region ★★★★
   CT scan of head ★★
   Visual evoked potentials ★★
   Auditory evoked potentials ★★

2. Intramedullary spinal tumour ★★★★
   Syringomyelia ★★★★
   Multiple sclerosis ★★★★
   Hereditary spastic paraplegia ★★
   Vascular/anatomical abnormality related to the scoliosis ★★
   Arnold-Chiari malformation with hydrocephalus ★★
   Subacute combined degeneration of the spinal cord ★
   There is sacral sparing of sensation to pin prick, suggesting an intramedullary lesion.

Case V

Bilateral neuralgic amyotrophy ★★★★
Inflammatory polyradiculopathy ★★
Traction injury to brachial plexus 0
Neuralgic amyotrophy is a disorder of unknown aetiology, although antecedent needle injections into the shoulder musculature and intercurrent infections have been suggested as possible aetiological factors. The disorder begins with aching pain in the lateral aspect of the shoulder, less often in the elbow or arm. Muscle weakness may develop within hours or days, and atrophy follows. Sensory loss is usually minimal and restricted to a small patch in the cutaneous distribution of the axillary nerve. Recovery usually takes several months and may not be complete for years. The CSF is normal.

ANSWERS TO DATA INTERPRETATIONS

1. Left anterior hemiblock ★★★★
   Incomplete right bundle branch block ★★★★
   Poor R-wave progression across chest leads ★★★★
   Borderline first degree heart block ★★

2. Otosclerosis ★★★★
   Middle ear disease ★
   Glue ear ★
   There is conductive deafness in both ears. 'Carhart's' notches are present in the bone conduction tracing at 2000 H_3. This has been ascribed to reduced inner ear hydrodynamics. With successful stapedectomy, the audiogram will normalise.

3. Atrial flutter with variable block ★★★★
   Atrial fibrillation 0

4. (a) Blood cultures ★★★★
       Anaerobic culture of synovial fluid ★★★★
       Vaginal/rectal/urethral swab for GC ★★★★
       Urine culture ★★★★
       Rheumatoid factor ★★
   (b) Septic arthritis ★★★★
       Gonococcal (GC) arthritis ★★★★
       Acute rheumatoid joint ★★★★
   Normal synovial fluid may have 13–180 cells/mm³, with mean monocyte count of 48% and mean lymphocyte count of 25%. Protein content is 0.45–2.7g/dl, with 63% albumin. Glucose and uric acid content is approximately the same as in serum. Rheumatoid synovial fluid is usually turbid with reduced

viscosity, increased protein content, and slight reduction of glucose levels relative to the blood. Leucocyte counts (predominantly polymorphonuclear cells) vary between a few thousand and more than 50,000 cells/mm³. Complement is usually reduced. In septic arthritis, leucocyte counts well in excess of 50,000/mm³ occur, and glucose content is significantly reduced.

5. (a) Excludes Epstein-Barr virus infection ★★★★
   (b) Cytomegalovirus infection ★★★★
       Toxoplasmosis ★★★★
   Interpretation of the heterophil antibody test:
   Infectious mononucleosis heterophil antibodies are removed by ox red cells, but not by guinea pig kidney cells.
   Heterophil antibodies present in normal serum are absorbed by guinea pig kidney, but not by ox erythrocytes.
   Heterophil antibodies in patients with serum sickness are absorbed by both antigens.

6. Thrombotic thrombocytopenic purpura (TTP) ★★★★
   Systemic lupus erythematosus ★★★★
   Collagen disease ★★★★
   Acute post-streptococcal glomerulonephritis ★★
   Carcinomatosis ★★
   TTP (Moschkovitz syndrome) is characterised by a microangiopathic haemolytic anaemia with thrombocytopenia, neurological signs, renal disease and fever. Renal disease is due to hyaline occlusion of capillaries and arterioles, and proliferative changes within the glomeruli. Typically, the blood film shows reticulocytosis and the presence of normoblasts, and characteristically schistocytes (fragmented cells). The antiglobulin test is negative. Thrombocytopenia is invariable. Bleeding time is prolonged. There is usually no evidence of DIC. A leucocytosis and 'left shift' may occur.

7. (a) Double-stranded DNA ★★★★
       TPHA ★★★★
       Complement levels ★★★★
       FTA Abs ★★★★
       CRP (C-reactive protein) ★★
   (b) SLE ★★★★
       Viral arthralgia (reactive) ★★★★
       Syphilis ★
   Acute 'false-positive' VDRL tests occur rarely in atypical pneumonia, and viral and bacterial infections. Chronic 'false positive' VDRL tests are associated with autoimmune diseases such as SLE, in narcotic addicts, leprosy and old age.

8. (a) Metabolic acidosis plus metabolic alkalosis ★★★★
       Metabolic acidosis ★
       Respiratory acidosis 0
   (b) Chronic renal failure and severe vomiting ★★★★
       Chronic renal failure and bicarbonate infusion ★★★★

9. Mixed respiratory alkalosis and metabolic acidosis ★★★★
   Respiratory alkalosis ★
   Hyperchloraemic acidosis 0
   Accumulated ammonia and progesterone, acting in concert with existing hypoxia and diaphragmatic displacement from ascites frequently cause patients with cirrhosis to demonstrate respiratory alkalosis. Diarrhoea is a cause of hyperchloraemic acidosis in cirrhosis, and in this case it has become superimposed in a pre existing respiratory alkalosis.

10. (a) Inappropriate ADH secretion ★★★★
    (b) Ca bronchus with ADH production ★★★★
        Head injury ★★
        Hypothyroidism ★★★★
        Pulmonary tuberculosis ★

Paper 3

Slide Interpretations

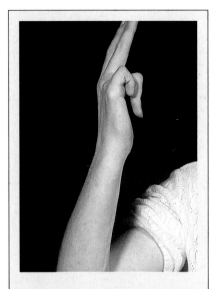

1. Suggest two possible causes for this appearance.

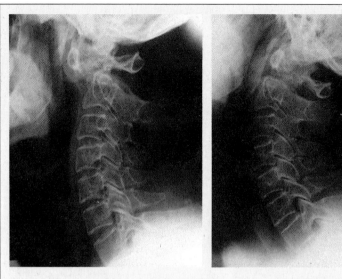

2. What abnormality is present on these X-rays? Give two possible causes.

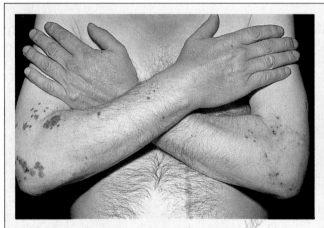

3. This man has similar lesions on his feet. What is the most probable diagnosis?

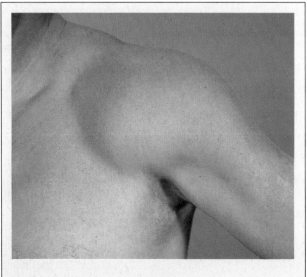

4. What is the most probable diagnosis?

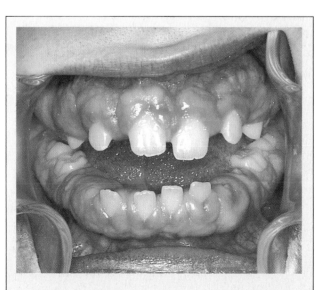

5. These are the gums of a 15-year-old. There was a family history of this condition. What is the most likely diagnosis?

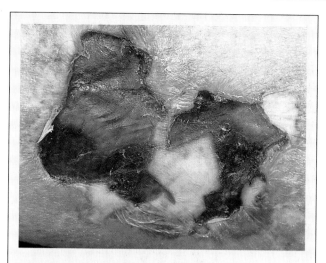

6. This man was suffering from myeloma.
   What lesion is shown?

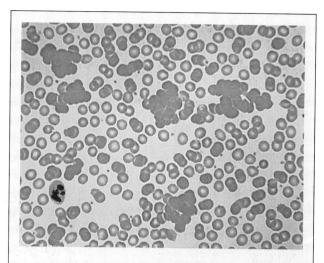

7. This is the blood film of a patient who complained of
   painful purple hands in the cold.
   List two conditions in which this appearance may be
   observed.

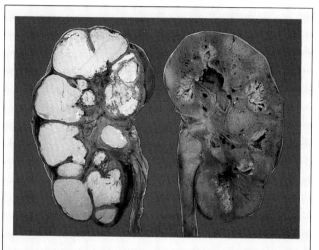

8. What is the diagnosis?

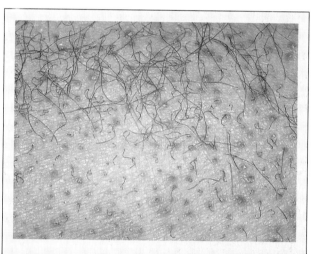

9. What is the likely diagnosis?

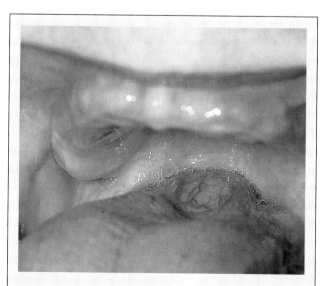

10. This mass on the back of the tongue had always been
    present in this patient.
    What is the likely diagnosis?

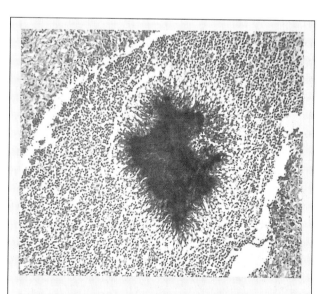

11. This tissue was present in an appendicectomy
    specimen.
    What is the most likely diagnosis?

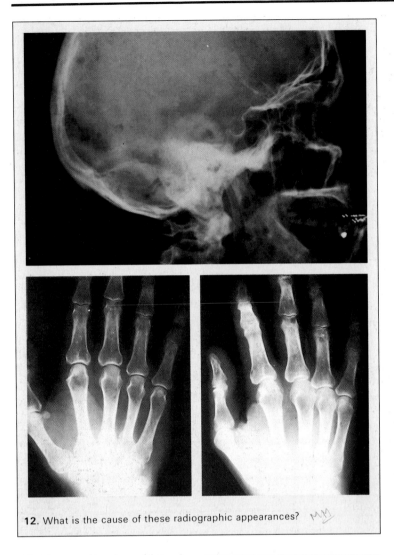

12. What is the cause of these radiographic appearances?

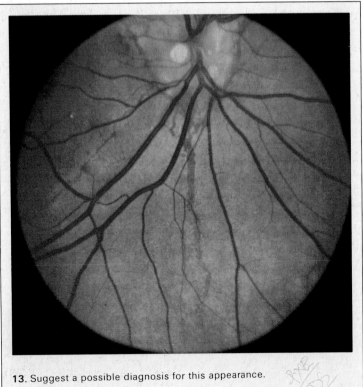

13. Suggest a possible diagnosis for this appearance.

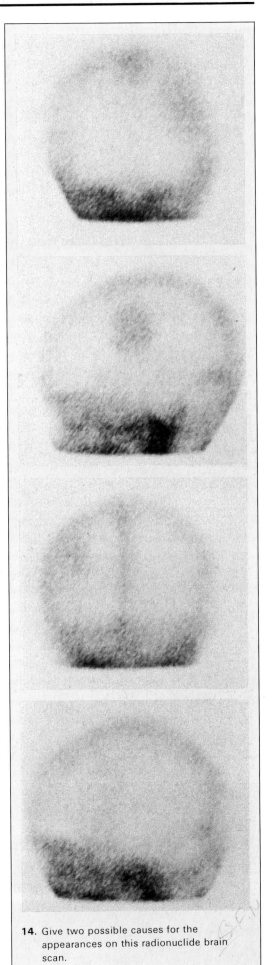

14. Give two possible causes for the appearances on this radionuclide brain scan.

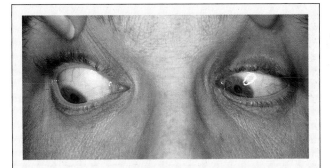

15. This patient is attempting to gaze downwards and to the right.
Suggest the most likely diagnosis.

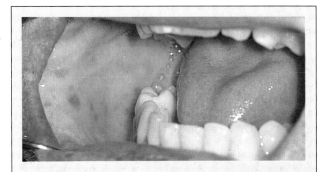

16. What is the most likely cause of this appearance?

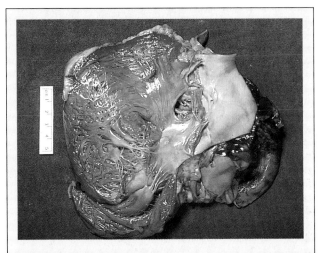

17. What lesion is visible in this heart?

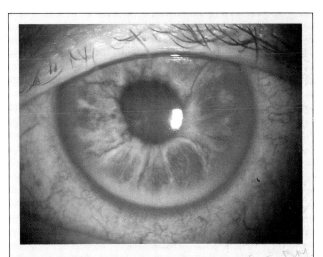

18. What is the most probable diagnosis?

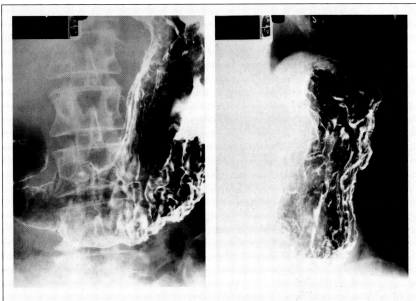

19. This is the barium meal of a patient complaining of severe weight loss and night sweats.
Suggest a possible cause for these radiographic appearances.

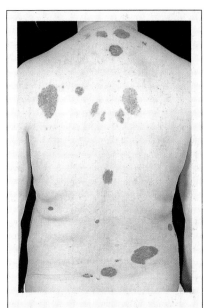

20. This 65-year-old man had received prolonged treatment with a 'tonic' 35 years ago. The lesions on his back appeared over a period of several years, and were progressively enlarging and firm.
What is the likely diagnosis?

Case Histories

CASE I

A 35-year-old woman farmer was admitted to hospital for investigation of headaches and visual loss. She had been in good health in the past, apart from an appendicectomy operation carried out ten years before. Her symptoms had started two years before with intermittent attacks of bitemporal headaches which were partially relieved by taking paracetamol. They were not associated with visual auras, nor teichopsia. For the past six months the headaches had become more frequent, and finally (over the preceding two months) they were present virtually daily, occasionally extending from the bitemporal region to the vertex of the skull. There was no associated vomiting. Three weeks before the patient had noticed that, while driving a tractor on her farm, she was tending to run into objects to the right. She also complained of a recent onset of difficulty in reading small print newspapers. Her menarche had taken place at 11 years of age, with regular periods at 4/28 until 18 months before, when they became less regular and more scanty. Over four months she thought that her concentration had diminished somewhat, and that she was feeling the cold more than previously.

On examination, she was a well-looking woman, if slightly pale. She was not icteric. Pulse 60/min regular, weight 62kg, blood pressure 130/70mmHg. Examination of the heart and lungs was normal. Examination of the breast revealed a trace of galactorrhoea on the left side. There was no abnormality in the abdomen, and pelvic examination was unremarkable. In the central nervous system there appeared to be a bitemporal upper quadrantic defect to red pin, and her visual acuity was 6/12 in both eyes. There was no abnormality on examination of the fundi. Tone and coordination reflexes were otherwise entirely normal.

Investigations

HAEMATOLOGY
Hb: 11.6g/dl (11.6g/100ml); WBC: 6.4×10^9/l (6,400/mm^3); Platelets: 235×10^9/l (235,000/mm^3).

BIOCHEMISTRY & SPECIAL INVESTIGATIONS
Urea: 6.4mmol/l (39mg/100ml); Sodium: 129mmol/l (129mEq/l); Potassium: 4.6mmol/l (4.6mEq/l); Chloride: 89mmol/l (89mEq/l); Bicarbonate: 27mmol/l (27mEq/l); Bilirubin: 16μmol/l (0.98mg/100ml); Alkaline phosphatase: 67iu/l (8.7KAU/100ml); Albumin: 40g/l (4.0g/100ml); Calcium: 2.4mmol/l (9.4mg/100ml); Phosphate: 0.98mmol/l (3.1mg/100ml); Luteinising hormone (LH): 2.6u/l (normal range: 3–9); Follicle stimulating hormone (FSH): 1.4u/l (normal range: 2–7); Oestradiol: 165pmol/l; Sex hormone binding globulin (SHBG): 47nmol/l (normal range: 38–103); T4: 46μmol/l (normal range: 58–174); Free thyroxine index (FTI): 48nmol/l (normal range: 58–174); Urinanalysis: normal.

1. List three mandatory investigations.

2. Give the most probable diagnosis.

CASE II

A 65-year-old man of no fixed abode was admitted in a drowsy state and hyperventilating. The only history available was from a friend who said that, over the previous week, he had been drinking heavily and three days before had experienced severe central chest pain which lasted about three hours and was associated with vomiting. Since that time, he had been a little breathless with moderate exertion, but had continued to drink alcohol.

On examination, he looked unkempt but was not anaemic or clubbed. Temperature was 37.5°C. There was no lymphadenopathy. Pulse was 120/min regular with a full volume, and blood pressure was 110/50mmHg. His limbs were warm. Cardiac auscultation revealed a fourth heart sound best heard at the apex, and basal crackles were present in both lung fields. All pulses were present. In the abdomen, the liver was smooth and enlarged by four centimetres. There was sparsity of hair; testes were normal in size, but soft. The patient was very drowsy, gave monosyllabic answers to questions and was disorientated in time and place. However, examination of the cranial nerves and peripheral nervous systems was otherwise unremarkable, except for diminished ankle jerks bilaterally. Both plantar responses were flexor.

Investigations

HAEMATOLOGY
Hb: 15.4g/dl (15.4g/100ml); MVC: 102fl (102μm^3); WBC: 14.8×10^9/l (14,800/mm^3); Neutrophils: 83%; Lymphocytes: 12%; Platelets: 167×10^9/l (167,000/mm^3).

BIOCHEMISTRY & SPECIAL INVESTIGATIONS
Blood glucose: 3.8mmol/l (68mg/100ml); Urea: 7.6mmol/l (46mg/100ml); Creatinine: 0.13mmol/l (1.47mg/100ml); Sodium: 134mmol/l (134 mEq/l); Potassium: 4mmol/l (4mEq/l); Chloride: 98mmol/l (98mEq/l); Bicarbonate: 12mmol/l (12mEq/l); Bilirubin: 28μmol/l (1.65mg/100ml); Alkaline phosphatase: 76iu/l (9.9KAU/100ml); Total protein: 67g/l (6.7g/100ml); Albumin: 35g/l (3.5g/100ml); Calcium: 2.1mmol/l (8.2mg/100ml); Phosphate: 0.7mmol/l (2.2mg/100ml); Serum glutamic oxaloacetic transaminase (SGOT): 56iu/l; CXR: normal; Urinanalysis: urine ketones negative; Blood cultures: negative after 24 h growth.

1. List three investigations which would be considered essential in the patient's immediate management.

2. List three probable underlying diagnoses.

CASE III

A 34-year-old vegan (strict vegetarian) woman presented with a four-week history of insomnia and loss of appetite. For two weeks she had been vomiting, and had lost 6 lbs in weight. One week before the patient had developed soreness in her joints, particularly the knees and ankles, and complained of a persistent feeling of irritation in her lungs. She would cough in an attempt to clear this, but would not bring up any sputum. All her symptoms had developed since the birth of her second child, 5 weeks before. During her pregnancy she had been in good health, and had taken vitamin preparations to supplement her diet. In her family history, an aunt had undergone surgery to the neck because of calcium problems.

On examination, her affect was flat but she was not anaemic or clubbed. Temperature 37°C, pulse 86/min regular, blood pressure 140/100mmHg. Heart and lungs were normal. There was no lymphadenopathy. In the abdomen, there was no enlargement of liver, spleen or kidneys, but striae gravidarum were present. Pelvic examination was unremarkable. There were no neurological abnormalities, and fundi were normal.

HAEMATOLOGY
Hb: 11.6g/dl (11.6g/100ml); WBC: 6.4 × 10⁹/l (6,400/mm³); Normal differential count; Platelets: 246 × 10⁹/l (246,000/mm³); ESR: 68mm/h.

BIOCHEMISTRY
Urea: 9.2mmol/l (56mg/100ml); Creatinine: 0.1mmol/l (1.13mg/100ml); Sodium: 138mmol/l (138mEq/l); Potassium: 4.2mmol/l (4.2mEq/l); Chloride: 96mmol/l (96mEq/l); Bicarbonate: 24mmol/l (24mEq/l); Bilirubin: 16μmol/l (1.3mg/100ml); Alkaline phosphatase: 133iu/l (17.3KAU/100ml); Total protein: 72g/l (7.2g/100ml); Albumin: 34g/l (3.4g/100ml); Calcium: 2.99mmol/l (11.72mg/100ml); Phosphate: 1.36mmol/l (4.4mg/100ml); Urinanalysis: normal.

RADIOLOGY
CXR: Slight bilateral hilar enlargement – follow-up film advised; ECG: first degree heart block, normal QRS axis, no repolarisation abnormalities.

1. Suggest two investigations which would be diagnostically useful.

2. Suggest a likely diagnosis.

CASE IV

A 21-year-old woman presented with a three-day history of clumsiness of her hands and episodes of double vision. She had developed a strange sensation on the right side of the face, and on the morning of admission had started to vomit. On the day prior to the start of her first symptoms, the patient had been a passenger in a car involved in a head-on collision. She had apparently suffered no injuries of note, and had not lost consciousness. She had been well in the past, and was on oral contraceptives. There was no family history of note, and the patient was taking no other drugs.

On examination she was alert and not anaemic, nor clubbed. Cardiovascular, respiratory and abdominal examinations were unremarkable. Pulse 86/min regular, blood pressure 120/70mmHg. Her speech appeared slurred, and she was tilting her head to the right. She seemed to have diplopia in all directions of gaze, with inability to adduct the left eye and abduct the right eye. Both horizontal and vertical nystagmus was present, and the right side of the face appeared weak. She also seemed to have decreased hearing on the right. There was impaired pin-prick sensation and light touch sensation over the entire right side of the body, and the corneal reflex was absent on the right. Reflexes appeared increased in the left arm and leg, and left ankle clonus was present. There was a left extensor plantar response. The patient seemed to fall to the left on standing up, and was unable to walk very far without assistance.

Hb: 13.2g/dl (13.2g/100ml); WBC: 6.8 × 10⁹/l (6,800/mm³); ESR: 6 mm/h; Urea and electrolytes: normal; Liver function tests: normal; Urinanalysis: normal; CXR: lungs clear, heart size normal.

1. List two investigations which would assist in obtaining a diagnosis.

2. Give two possible underlying diagnoses.

CASE V

A 32-year-old school teacher was admitted with a three-week history of a dry cough, loss of appetite and increasing shortness of breath. He had had intermittent headaches for a week, and six days before admission he complained of pain in the lower back region, worse on coughing, as well as of weakness and paraesthesiae affecting the legs and arms. These symptoms progressed over the ensuing days, and became so severe that the patient was too weak to stand. On the day before admission he had become incontinent of urine.

On examination, he appeared dehydrated with a temperature of 37°C. Pulse 115/min, blood pressure 105/80mmHg. Examination of the heart was normal, but there were some crackles over his right mid and lower zones. There was no bronchial breathing. The abdomen was normal. Examination of the central nervous system revealed weakness affecting the legs and arms. His biceps jerk was present, but all other reflexes were absent. Pin-prick sensation and light touch were absent below a demarkation level of T2. Examination of the cranial nerves was unremarkable, and fundoscopy was normal. The patient was unable to void urine when asked to, and approximately twelve hours after admission there was urinary retention.

HAEMATOLOGY
Hb: 16.5g/dl (16.5g/100ml); MCV: 94fl (94μm³); WBC: 21 × 10⁹/l (21,000/mm³); Neutrophils: 82%; Lymphocytes: 8 × 10⁹/l (8,000/mm³).

BIOCHEMISTRY & RADIOLOGY
Urea: 14.6mmol/l (80mg/100ml); Sodium: 145mmol/l (145mEq/l); Potassium: 3.8mmol/l (3.8mEq/l); Chloride: 108mmol/l (108mEq/l); Bicarbonate: 23mmol/l (23mEq/l); Bilirubin: 22μmol/l (1.3mg/100ml); Alkaline phosphatase: 58iu/l (6KAU/100ml); Albumin: 37g/l (3.7g/100ml); CSF examination: protein 0.6g/l (60mg/100ml); Glucose: 4.2mmol/l (76mg/100ml); Simultaneous blood glucose: 5.8mmol/l (100mg/100ml); Cytology: 4 lymphocytes/mm³. CXR: a patchy infiltrate is present in the right mid and lower zones; Heart size normal.

1. List four investigations which would assist in the patient's immediate management.

2. Suggest two possible diagnoses.

Data Interpretations

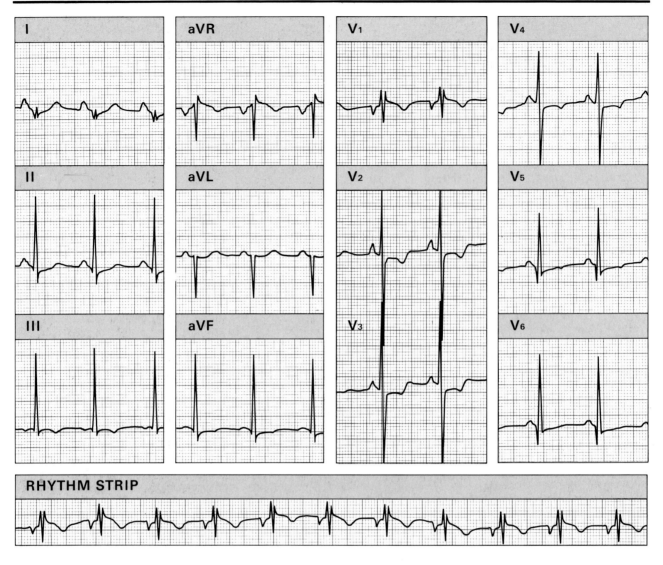

1. This is the ECG of a 30-year-old woman with recurrent syncopal attacks.
   (a) List three abnormalities. (b) Suggest a possible underlying diagnosis.

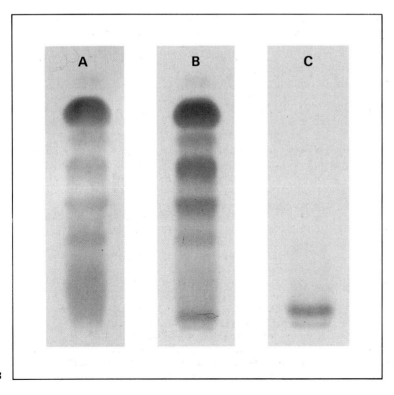

2. **A** represents the serum electrophoretic strip from a normal person; **B** is the serum from a patient with a pathological fracture, and **C** is the electrophoretic strip from his urine. What is the most likely diagnosis?

3.8

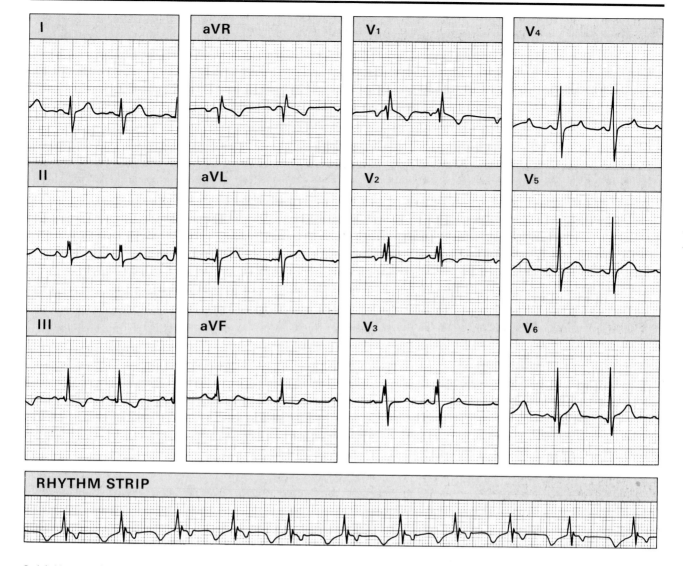

I	aVR	V₁	V₄
II	aVL	V₂	V₅
III	aVF	V₃	V₆

RHYTHM STRIP

3. **(a)** List two abnormalities. **(b)** What is the likely diagnosis? **(c)** List two associated auscultatory abnormalities.

4. A 56-year-old man becomes breathless and hypotensive (95/70mmHg), 72 hours following a lobectomy for carcinoma.
Blood gases: PaO_2: 7.4kPa (56mmHg); $PaCO_2$: 3.9kPa (30mmHg); pH: 7.43.
Suggest two possible causes for these findings.

5. A 35-year-old pump attendant is investigated for recurrent haemoptyses over a two-month period.
Hb: 7.2g/dl (7.2g/100ml); MCV: 76fl ($76\mu m^3$); Urea: 18mmol/l; (115mg/dl); Urine microscopy: red cells +++; CXR: confluent alveolar shadows.
(a) Suggest two diagnostically useful investigations.
(b) What is the most likely diagnosis?

6. A 64-year-old long-standing alcoholic patient is admitted following an episode of amaurosis fugax. On examination, an enlarged irregular liver is present, and peripheral oedema is abundant.
Hb: 19.6g/dl (19.6g/100ml); PCV: 0.58 (58%); MCV: 102fl ($102\mu m^3$); Platelets: 88×10^9/l (88,000/mm^3); Albumin: 20g/l (2.0g/100ml).
(a) List four diagnostically useful investigations.
(b) Give a unifying diagnosis.

7. A 14-year-old girl, known to suffer from beta-thalassaemia major, is admitted for treatment of heart failure. She is noted to have a greyish appearance.

Hb: 7.8g/dl (7.8g/100ml); Fe: $32\mu mol/l$; TIBC: $34\mu mol/l$.
Give two possible causes for her heart failure.

8. An 18-year-old girl gives a long history of abdominal pain, nausea and drowsiness after drinking fruit juice. Thirty minutes after consuming 150ml of fruit juice, her blood glucose has fallen to 2.1mmol/l.
(a) What is the likely underlying diagnosis?
(b) What investigation will confirm the diagnosis?

9. A 58-year-old man is receiving antidysrhythmic treatment following a myocardial infarction. A goitre is noted.
T4: 212nmol/l (normal range 58–174); THUT: 93 (normal range 92–118); FTI: 188 (normal range 58–174); T3: 1.88nmol/l (normal range 1.23–3.07).
(a) Suggest a cause for the above thyroid function tests.
(b) What further investigation is most useful?

10. A 36-year-old woman is investigated for severe hirsuties, oligomenorrhoea and obesity.
9a.m. cortisol: 480nmol/l ($16\mu g$/100ml); 9a.m. testosterone: 5.6nmol/l(normal range: 0.8–3.1); LH: 7.2iu/l; FSH: 2.8iu/l; Prolactin: 380mU/l(normal range: <360); SHBG: 22nmol/l (normal range: 46-110).
After 0.5mg dexamethasone 6-hourly for 48 hours:
9a.m. cortisol: <70nmol/l; 9a.m. testosterone: 5.3nmol/l.
(a) What two further investigations are indicated?
(b) What is the most likely diagnosis?

3.9

Answers

1. Dupuytren's contracture ★★★
   Ulnar nerve lesion ★★
   Burns' contracture ★

2. (a) Atlanto-axial subluxation ★★★★
   (b) Rheumatoid arthritis ★★★★
       Psoriatic arthropathy ★★★★
       Still's disease ★★★★
       Ankylosing spondylitis ★★★
       Systemic lupus erythematosus ★★★
       Trauma ★★★
   These flexion/extension views show gross subluxation.

3. Henoch-Schoenlein purpura ★★★★
   Anaphylactoid purpura ★★★★
   Allergic vasculitis ★★★★
   Vasculitis ★★
   The rash of H-S purpura is initially urticarial, and gradually becomes haemorrhagic. The rash typically occurs in recurrent crops and may involve the face. This allergic vasculitis occurs most frequently after a streptococcal infection or occasionally after ingestion of a sensitising drug.

4. Large effusion in the shoulder joint ★★★★
   Bursitis 0
   In this case, this was caused by rheumatoid arthritis.

5. Familial gingival fibromatosis ★★★★
   Phenytoin-induced gum hyperplasia 0

6. Bullous pyoderma gangrenosum ★★★★
   Skin infarct ★★★★
   Vasculitis ★★★★
   Cryoglobulinaemia ★★★★
   Other associations of pyoderma gangrenosum include: Inflammatory bowel disease; Wegener's granulomatosis; Rheumatoid arthritis.

7. Cold agglutination disease ★★★★
   Mycoplasma pneumoniae ★★★★
   Infectious mononucleosis ★★★★
   Cytomegalovirus infection ★★★★
   Lymphoma ★★★★
   Perniosis 0
   Raynaud's phenomenon 0
   The cold agglutination syndrome is usually caused by IgM antibodies, which react at low temperatures to agglutinate red cells. Clinically, this may manifest as intravascular agglutination or a complement-dependent haemolytic anaemia. Upon exposure to cold, patients may note that hands, ears, nose or feet may turn purple and become painful; this process is rapidly reversed upon rewarming, and is distinguished from Raynaud's phenomenon in that there is no blanching phase and little evidence of hyperaemia.

8. Tuberculosis of the kidney ★★★★
   Renal adenocarcinoma 0
   Nephrolithiasis 0

9. Scurvy ★★★★
   Perifollicular haemorrhage ★
   Hyperkeratotic hair follicle ★
   Perifollicular haemorrhage, with hyperkeratotic hair follicles, is one of the earliest and most distinctive features of scurvy, appearing particularly on the posterior thighs, anterior forearms and abdomen. The hairs also become fragmented and coiled ('corkscrew hairs').

10. Lingual thyroid ★★★★
    Retropharyngeal mass ★
    This is usually associated with euthyroidism.

11. Actinomycosis ★★★★
    Mycotic abscess ★★
    Caused by *Actinomyces israelii*, the stained sulphur granule shown is composed of Gram-positive branching of often beaded 0.5–1.0μ filaments. This bacterium is sensitive to penicillin.

12. Multiple myeloma ★★★★
    Metastatic deposits ★
    Hyperparathyroidism 0
    The typical 'punched out' (i.e. osteolytic) lesions of multiple myeloma are shown. The skull, jaw, spine, ribs, clavicles, sternum and pelvis generally exhibit the greatest destruction, but any part of the skeleton including the phalanges, as shown here, may be involved. Osteoblastic reaction is extremely rare.

13. Angioid streaks ★★★★
    Neovascularisation of retina 0
    Retinal haemorrhage 0
    Angioid streaks underlie the retinal vessels and cross the fundus radially from the optic disc. They represent breaks in the elastic tissue of Bruch's membrane, and are found in:
    Pseudoxanthoma elasticum;
    Sickle cell disease;
    Ehlers-Danlos syndrome;
    Paget's disease.

14. Cerebral tumour ★★★★
    Meningioma ★★★★
    A–V malformation ★★
    Subdural haematoma 0

15. Left superior oblique palsy ★★★★
    Oculomotor palsy 0
    Left inferior oblique palsy 0
    There is incomplete depression of the adducted left eye on attempted downward gaze to the right.

16. Peutz-Jegher's syndrome ★★★★
    Addison's disease 0
    This is associated with hamartomatous polyps in the jejunum and ileum; gastric polyps (in 25% of cases), colorectal polyps (in 30–50% of cases) and benign ovarian tumours also occur. Malignancy tends to occur proximal to the ligament of Trietz. Both the melanin deposits shown as well as the associated polyps are transmitted by a single mendelian dominant trait.

17. Ventricular septal defect ★★★★
    Atrial septal defect 0
    Papillary muscle necrosis 0

18. Rubeotic glaucoma ★★★★
    Glaucoma ★★
    Rubeosis iridis ★★
    This is most commonly associated with retinal neovascularisation in diabetes mellitus. The neovascularisation occurs in the ciliary body and iris, leading to occlusion of the outflow tract, resulting in open-angle neovascular glaucoma, or to haemorrhagic glaucoma after rupture of a vessel. The hazy appearance of the cornea together with the irregular pupil are typical of glaucoma.

19. Gastric lymphoma ★★★★
    Ménétriér's disease ★★
    Gastric carcinoma ★★
    Symptoms of gastric lymphoma are similar to those of carcinoma except that some patients have a history similar to that of peptic ulcer, sometimes for several years. Reticulum cell sarcoma and lymphosarcoma are the most common types, and exfoliative cytology is positive in up to 90% of patients.

20. Multiple squamous carcinomata secondary to arsenic
    intake ★★★★
    Psoriasis 0
    Pigmentation and scaling of the skin, hyperkeratosis of palms
    and soles, transverse white lines of fingernails (Mee's lines) and
    perforation of the nasal septum are important cutaneous
    manifestations of chronic arsenic poisoning. Arsenical
    hyperkeratotic lesions may undergo malignant change (Bowen's
    disease).

ANSWERS TO CASE HISTORIES

Case I

1. 9 a.m. cortisol ★★★★
    Skull X-ray ★★★★
    Coned view of pituitary fossa ★★★★
    CT scan of hypothalamus and pituitary ★★★★
    Prolactin estimation ★★★★
    Formal perimetry ★★★★
    Dynamic testing of pituitary function ★★
    Plasma and urine osmolality estimation ★★
    Visual evoked potentials ★★
    CSF examination 0

2. Pituitary adenoma ★★★★
    Prolactinoma ★★★★
    Hypopituitarism ★
    The presence of inappropriately low gonadotrophins in the
    presence of a low oestradiol level suggests hypothalamic/pituitary
    disease. The presence of galactorrhoea suggests that a
    prolactinoma might be present.

Case II

1. Serum lactic acid ★★★★
    Arterial blood gases ★★★★
    Electrocardiogram ★★★★
    Serum amylase ★★★★
    Cardiac enzymes ★★★★
    CT scan of head ★★
    Salicylate estimation ★★

2. Lactic acidosis ★★★★
    Metabolic acidosis secondary to methanol consumption ★★★★
    Myocardial infarction ★★★★
    Pulmonary oedema ★★★★
    Ethylene glycol poisoning ★★
    Thiamine deficiency ★
    The presence of a large anion gap (28mmol/l) should suggest the
    presence of lactic acidosis. Possible precipitating causes in this
    case include circulatory failure, and possible ingestion of
    methanol.

Case III

1. Bronchoscopy with bronchial brushings and transbronchial lung
    biopsy ★★★★
    Liver biopsy ★★★★
    Mediastinoscopy with biopsy ★★
    Bone marrow aspirate for culture of AAFB ★★
    Early morning urine for AAFB ★★
    Mantoux test ★★
    Serum angiotensin converting enzyme level ★★
    CT scan of lungs ★★
    Protein electrophoresis ★★
    Carbon monoxide transfer factor ★★
    1,25 dihydroxycholecalciferol ★
    24 h urinary calcium ★

2. Tuberculosis ★★★★
    Sarcoidosis ★★★★

Vitamin D intoxication ★
The findings would be compatible with either sarcoidosis or
tuberculosis. It is therefore essential to obtain a tissue diagnosis.

Case IV

1. Contrast enhanced CT scan ★★★★
    Vertebral angiogram ★★★★
    Magnetic resonance imaging of brainstem ★★★★
    Blood glucose ★
    EEG 0

2. Brainstem cerebrovascular accident ★★★★
    Vertebral artery dissection ★★★★
    Vertebral artery embolism ★★★★
    Episode of multiple sclerosis ★★★★
    Traumatic pontine haematoma ★★
    The patient has a brainstem syndrome. In the presence of full
    consciousness, a brainstem syndrome secondary to a subdural
    haematoma is very unlikely.

Case V

1. Myelogram ★★★★
    Sagittal magnetic resonance imaging of head/spine ★★★★
    Spinal X-rays ★★★★
    Mycoplasma pneumoniae titres ★★★★
    Anti-nuclear factor ★★
    Sputum culture ★★
    Blood gases ★★
    CSF for oligoclonal bands ★★
    Blood cultures ★★
    EEG ★★
    Nerve conduction studies ★

2. Parainfectious transverse myelitis ★★★★
    Transverse myelitis ★★★★
    Multiple sclerosis ★★★★
    Chest symptoms with mycoplasma pneumoniae may typically
    persist for three to six weeks. Non-respiratory complications
    include intravascular haemolysis (cold agglutinins), psychosis,
    meningitis, meningoencephalitis, neuropathy (Guillain-Barré
    syndrome), and cerebellar ataxia as part of the parainfectious
    syndrome.

ANSWERS TO DATA INTERPRETATIONS

1. (a) Left ventricular hypertrophy ★★★★
        Left ventricular hypertrophy with strain ★★★★
        Left atrial hypertrophy ★★★★
        Septal hypertrophy ★★★★
        Deep Q wave in V_5, V_6, aVL ★★★★

(b) Hypertrophic obstructive cardiomyopathy ★★★★
        Aortic stenosis ★★
        Ventricular septal defect 0
    The history of syncopal attacks is compatible with a diagnosis
    of HOCM. The ECG is most frequently associated with
    sinus rhythm and LVH. The occurrence of atrial fibrillation
    is an ominous sign because of the dependence of diastolic
    filling on atrial contraction. A short P–R interval with a δ wave is
    not uncommonly seen. The prominent Q waves in the V_5, V_6,
    aVL and Lead I have been ascribed to gross septal hypertrophy.

2. Myeloma ★★★★
    Paraproteinaemia ★★★★
    Cirrhosis 0
    A light chain 'M band' is shown both in the serum and in the
    urine, and there is reduced gamma globulin. These are the
    features of paraproteinaemia.

Answers

3.
(a) Incomplete right bundle branch block ★★★★
Right axis deviation ★★★★
Left atrial hypertrophy ★★
(b) Atrial septal defect ★★★★
Cor pulmonale ★★
(c) Fixed splitting of second sound ★★★★
Pulmonary ejection systolic murmur ★★★★
Tricuspid mid diastolic murmur ★★★★
Pulmonary regurgitation murmur ★★

When pulmonary hypertension has supervened, the pulmonary mid systolic flow murmur is replaced by a softer, shorter mid systolic murmur. Tricuspid flow murmurs then vanish.

4.
Pulmonary embolus ★★★★
Pneumothorax ★★★★
Myocardial infarction ★★
Pulmonary oedema ★★

If this was due to pulmonary oedema, the PO_2 would be much lower by the time hypotension had supervened.

5.
(a) Lung biopsy ★★★★
Renal biopsy ★★★★
Anti-glomerular membrane antibody ★★★★
Pulmonary CO transfer factor ★★
(b) Goodpasture's syndrome ★★★★

Patients with Goodpasture's syndrome have a circulating IgG antibody against a glycoprotein of both the glomerular membrane and lung basement membrane. In 50% of cases, the IgG fixes complement. The condition will result in severe necrosis of the glomerulus and pulmonary haemorrhage. The DLCO is increased because of alveolar haemorrhage.

6.
(a) PaO_2 ★★★★
Alpha-fetoprotein ★★★★
Liver ultrasound ★★★★
Liver CT scan ★★★★
Intravenous urogram ★★★★
(b) Cirrhosis with erythropoietin-secreting hepatoma ★★★★
Cirrhosis with secondary polycythaemia associated with pulmonary A–V shunting ★★★★

7.
Transfusion haemosiderosis ★★★★
Iron deposition in the myocardium ★★★★
Chronic anaemia ★★★★

Cardiac disease in β-thalassaemia major takes three forms: recurrent acute pericarditis, congestive cardiac failure, and cardiac arrhythmias. Iron deposition in the myocardium begins by the age of 5–6.

Haemosiderosis is largely the result of the many transfusions required to maintain life, but an additional factor is enhanced absorption of iron from the gastrointestinal tract. Typically, serum iron is elevated with increased saturation of the transferrin. Chelating agents, such as desferrioxamine mesylate, can lead to the removal of substantial amounts of iron.
The prognosis of patients with thalassaemia major is determined by the cardiac disease.

8.
(a) Hereditary fructose intolerance ★★★★
Galactosaemia 0
(b) Fructosuria and hypoglycaemia after oral or IV fructose administration ★★★★

Hereditary fructose intolerance is an autosomal recessive condition associated with a structural alteration of phosphofructoaldolase B. Affected subjects commonly note dyspepsia and anxiety with fructose ingestion, and usually avoid the offending food through personal observation.
Hypoglycaemia results from a marked decrease in glucose production by the liver shortly after fructose loading. The untreated infantile form is associated with vomiting, failure to grow, hypoglycaemia, jaundice, hepatosplenomegaly, ascites, aminoacidaemia, hyperuricaemia and acidosis, making the clinical presentation difficult to differentiate from galactosaemia

and tyrosinosis.

9.
(a) Amiodarone therapy ★★★★
Over-replacement with thyroxine and propranolol ★
(b) TRH test ★★★★
Basal (IRMA) TSH estimation ★★
Thyroid antibodies ★
Technetium scan of thyroid ★

These are typical thyroid function tests in a patient on amiodarone. The effects of this drug on thyroid function are complex and may be associated with hyperthyroidism (Jod-Basedow effect), euthyroidism, or hypothyroidism. Amiodarone blocks T4 to T3 conversion in the periphery (by blocking deiodinase activity); this results in a low T3 level but elevated T4. A TRH test is necessary to determine whether hyperthyroidism has occurred, a flat TSH response suggesting thyrotoxicosis. With florid clinical thyrotoxicosis on amiodarone, although the T4 and FTI may be massively elevated, the T3 while elevated is inappropriately low for the degree of thyrotoxicosis (because of blockage of T4 to T3 conversion).

10.
(a) Ovarian ultrasound ★★★★
Venous catheter to localise the origin of the abnormal androgen ★★★★
Laparotomy ★★
CT scan of pelvis ★
Skull X-ray 0.
(b) Ovarian androgen-secreting tumour ★★★★
Ovarian tumour ★★
Congenital adrenal hyperplasia 0

The failure of the testosterone to fall following a low dose dexamethasone suppression test indicates that this is not a case of polycystic ovaries or CAH. The most likely cause of this patient's symptoms is an androgen-secreting tumour, most probably ovarian in origin.

Paper 4

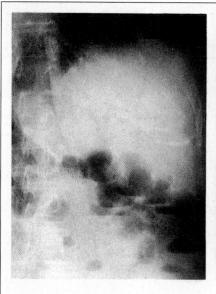

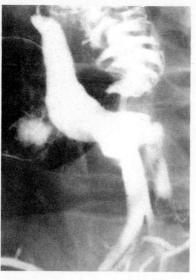

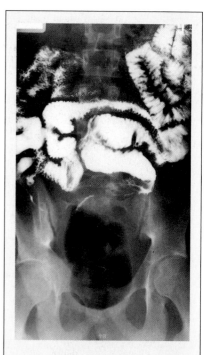

1. This patient had previously undergone an endoscopic procedure for removal of gallstones.
What abnormality is shown?

2. What is the most likely cause of this radiological appearance?

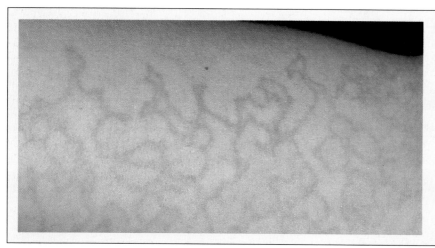

3. (a) What is this skin eruption?
   (b) What is the probable underlying condition?

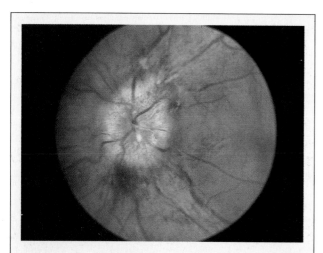

4. (a) What is the diagnosis?
   (b) List three possible causes.

5. This specimen was removed from a hypertensive patient as a curative procedure.
What lesion is shown?

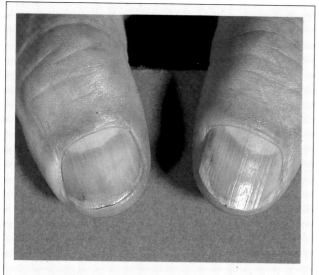

6. Suggest a possible cause for the appearance of these nails.

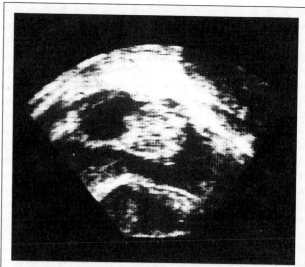

7. This is the echocardiogram of a patient who presented with cerebrovascular accident and had a high ESR. What is the diagnosis?

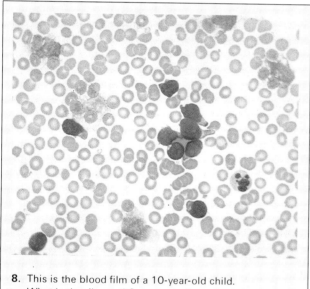

8. This is the blood film of a 10-year-old child. What is the diagnosis?

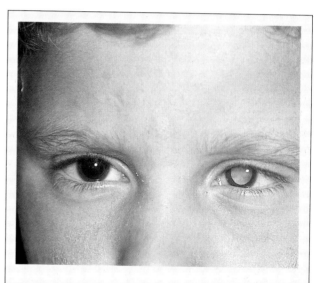

9. What is the most likely cause of this appearance?

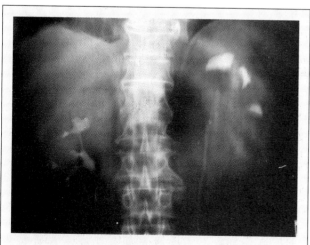

10. This investigation was undertaken to elucidate the cause of painless haematuria in a 48-year-old man. What is the most likely diagnosis?

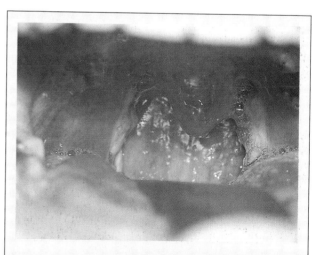

11. List two possible causes for this appearance of the fauces.

Slide Interpretations

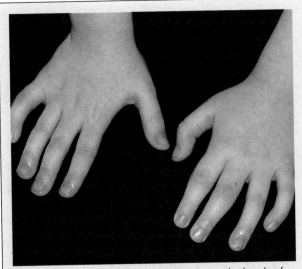

12. **(a)** What striking abnormality is seen on the hands of this 12-year-old child?
(b) What is the probable diagnosis?

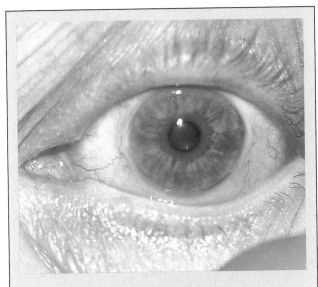

13. What underlying biochemical abnormality is likely to be present?

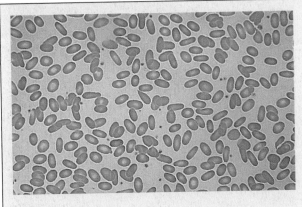

14. List two possible complications of the condition shown on this film.

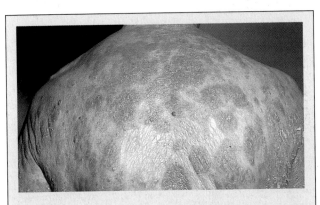

15. This pruritic papular eruption had been present for four months.
What is the diagnosis?

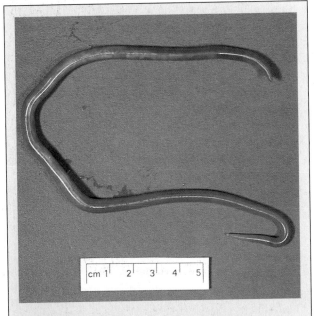

16. This worm was found in a patient's faeces.
List three complications of infestation with this worm.

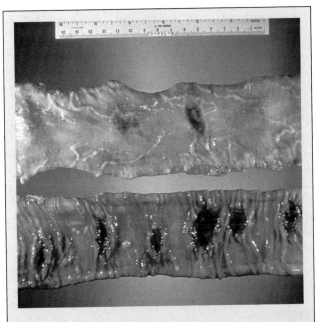

17. What is the cause of these ileal lesions?

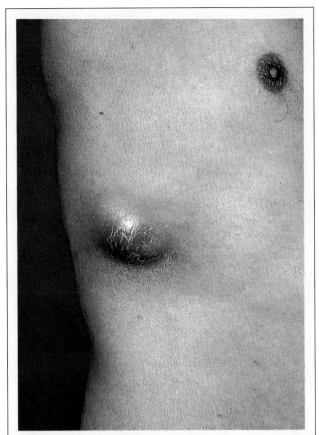

18. This lesion occurred insidiously, over a four week period. What is the most likely diagnosis?

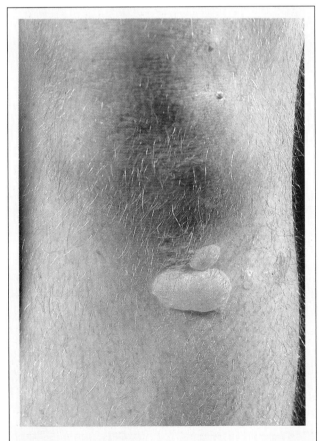

19. What is the diagnosis?

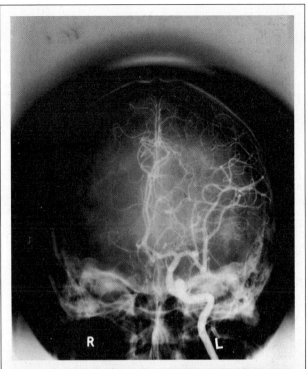

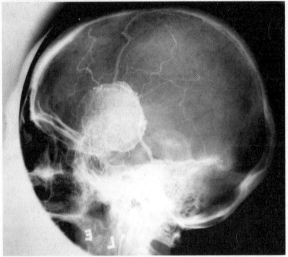

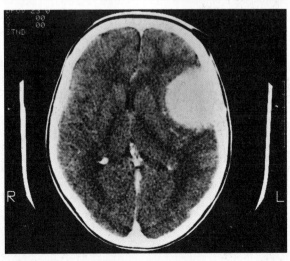

20. This carotid angiogram and contrast enhanced CT scan were carried out in a 45-year-old man with recent onset of right-sided Jacksonian seizures.
What is the most likely diagnosis?

An 8-year-old schoolboy was referred for assessment of tall stature and precocious sexual development. He was the product of a full-term normal vaginal delivery and had normal milestones for the first three years of life. At 18 months, he suffered from a bout of gastroenteritis with nausea and vomiting which lasted over three weeks, and required hospitalisation with intravenous fluid administration. At the age of three, his mother noticed that he was much taller than his peers and that a few wisps of pubic hair were present around the base of his penis. Over the ensuing two years, the shaft of the penis grew and his height was much more than either familial inheritance or age would justify.

On examination, he was a tall 8-year-old with greasy facial skin and hair. Muscle development was disproportionate to his age. There were a few wisps of axillary hair, and pubic hair consisted of between 40 and 100 hairs over 1 cm long at the base of the penis. Penile shaft corresponded to that expected in late puberty, but the testes were bilaterally 3 ml in volume and soft, and body segment measurements were approximately equal. The cardiovascular system was unremarkable, and blood pressure was 105/60mmHg (lying) and 105/60mmHg (standing). Abdominal and central nervous system examinations were unremarkable.

Investigations

HAEMATOLOGY
Hb: 12.6g/dl (12.6g/100ml); WBC: 6.4 × 10^9/l (6,400/mm³); ESR: 6mm/h.

BIOCHEMISTRY
Urea: 4.6mmol/l (28mg/100ml); Sodium: 136 mmol/l (136 mEq/l); Potassium: 5.1mmol/l (5.1mEq/l); Bicarbonate: 22mmol/l (22mEq/l); Chloride: 105 mmol/l (105mEq/l); Bilirubin: 16μmol/l (0.97mg/100ml); Alkaline phosphatase: 216iu/l (28KAU/100ml); Total proteins: 65g/l (6.5g/100ml); Calcium: 2.4mmol/l (9.4mg/100ml); Phosphate: 0.89mmol/l (2.9mg/100ml); 9a.m. cortisol: 188nmol/l (7.1μg/100ml) (normal range: 170–700nmol/l); Plasma renin activity: 6,400pmol/l/h (normal range: 230–1000pmol/l/h); Bone age: 11 years.

1. List three essential investigations which would assist in establishing the diagnosis.

2. Suggest the most likely diagnosis.

A 38-year-old man, not seen by his neighbours for two days, was found in a drowsy state in his flat. He was known to indulge in excessive alcohol consumption, and in the past had had several peptic ulcers with haematemeses. Recently, the patient had begun vomiting at frequent intervals, and had been referred to Surgical Outpatients where he was advised to undergo a partial gastrectomy because of pyloric stenosis.

On admission, he was disorientated, drowsy and cyanosed with inadequate respiratory movements. Temperature was 37.2°C, pulse 100/min and blood pressure 150/60mmHg. There was no lymphadenopathy, the trachea was central, and the lungs were clear. Heart sounds were normal. In the abdomen, three fingers of hepatomegaly was present, but the spleen was not palpable. The epigastrium seemed tender, with a small mass palpable to the right of the umbilicus. Rectal examination was unremarkable.

On neurological examination, corneal reflexes were depressed and gag reflexes impaired. His eye movements appeared dysconjugate, with first degree horizontal and vertical nystagmus. There appeared to be mild truncal and limb ataxia, but no neck stiffness. Reflexes were generally brisk, and both plantar reflexes were equivocal. A few hours after admission, the patient's level of consciousness appeared to deteriorate further, with his eyes maintaining a forward conjugate gaze with no spontaneous or doll's eye movements.

Investigations

HAEMATOLOGY
Hb: 14.6g/dl (14.6g/100ml); MCV: 104fl (104μm³); WBC: 12.6 × 10^9/l (12,600/mm³); Neutrophils: 75%; Platelets: 350 × 10^9/l (350,000/mm³); ESR: 3mm/h.

BIOCHEMISTRY
Urea: 13.2mmol/l (80mg/100ml); Creatinine: 0.11mmol/l (1.24mg/100ml); Sodium: 130mmol/l (130mEq/l); Potassium: 2.9mmol/l (2.9mEq/l); Bicarbonate: 27mmol/l (27mEq/l); Chloride: 87mmol/l (87mEq/l); Bilirubin: 20μmol/l (1.2mg/100ml); Alkaline phosphatase: 96iu/l (12.4KAU/100ml); Total protein: 66g/l (6.6g/100ml); Albumin: 34g/l (3.4g/100ml); Calcium: 2.06mmol/l (8mg/100ml); Phosphate: 0.6mmol/l (1.9mg/100ml); Serum glutamic oxaloacetic transaminase (SGOT): 36iu/l; Creatine kinase: 316iu/l; Gamma glutamyl transpeptidase: 147iu/l; Urinanalysis: normal; Arterial gases on 24% inspired oxygen; pH: 7.3; PaO$_2$: 10.4kPa (78mmHg); PaCO$_2$: 7.1kPa (53mmHg).

RADIOLOGY
CXR: normal; ECG: sinus tachycardia, U waves present in V$_1$ to V$_4$; CT brain scan: cortical atrophy present.

1. List three investigations which would assist in the patient's management.

2. What is the most likely diagnosis?

A 16-year-old previously fit schoolgirl was admitted to hospital for observation, following the onset of pain in the right hip. This had come on whilst she was playing sports at school, and was sufficiently severe that she felt unable to bear weight on the joint. She had been fit and well in the past, with no serious medical complaints and was on no medication. There was no family history of note.

On examination the patient was obviously distressed, but passive movements of her left hip seemed full, although inducing some pain. She was not anaemic. Pingueculae were noted in both eyes. Although 16, she was clearly delayed in her pubertal development, and had not as yet menstruated. Some pigmented areas were noted over the anterior chest wall. Abdominal examination revealed three fingers hepatomegaly and a 4cm spleen, neither of which was tender.

Hb: 11.4g/dl (11.4g/100ml); MCV: 88fl (88μm^3); WBC: 3.1 × 10^9/l (3,100/mm^3); Neutrophils: 68%; Lymphocytes: 24%; Platelets: 87 × 10^9/l (87,000/mm^3); ESR: 12mm/h; CXR: normal; X-ray of pelvis and hips: normal; Bone scan: compatible with a developing avascular necrosis of the femoral head.

1. List two investigations which would help in the patient's management.

2. Suggest two possible diagnoses.

CASE IV

A 36-year-old woman suffering from Down's syndrome was admitted for investigation for weight loss and abdominal swelling. She had been well until a year ago, when she complained of anorexia. Over the ensuing months, her mother noted gradual weight loss totalling 10kg. Three months before the patient complained of vague abdominal pains which were ascribed to irritable bowels by her GP. Despite a course of antispasmodic drugs, her symptoms failed to resolve and she was referred to hospital outpatients where she was noted to be pale and cachectic. In view of her history of occasional vomiting, a barium meal was organised which was normal. She was admitted following an emergency request by her doctor who had been called when she complained of generalised abdominal pain.

On admission she was noticed to be wasted and anaemic. She seemed drowsy. Pulse 102/min regular, blood pressure 100/60mmHg. Her jugular venous pulse was raised 3cm, but examination of her lungs was entirely normal. Heart sounds also appeared normal. Temperature was 37.4°C. There was no lymphadenopathy, but significant abdominal distension and a fluid thrill were present. Neither liver nor spleen was palpable, and pelvic examination was entirely unremarkable. Sigmoidoscopy was normal up to 15cm. There was no abnormality in the central nervous system.

Investigations

HAEMATOLOGY
Hb: 9.8g/dl (9.8g/100ml); MCV: 87fl (87μm^3); WBC: 6.4 × 10^9/l (6,400/mm^3); Blood film: normocytic normochromic; ESR: 62mm/h; Sodium: 132mmol/l (132mEq/l); Potassium: 4.1mmol/l (4.1mEq/l); Bicarbonate: 22mmol/l (22mEq/l); Chloride: 96mmol/l (96mEq/l); Urea: 5.6mmol/l (34mg/100ml); Creatinine: 0.09mmol/l (1.07mg/100ml); Bilirubin: 18μmol/l (1mg/100ml); Alkaline phosphatase: 176iu/l (23KAU/100ml); Total protein: 54g/l (5.4g/100ml); Albumin: 30g/l (3.0g/100ml); Calcium: 2.02mmol/l (8mg/100ml); Phosphate: 0.97mmol/l (3.5mg/100ml); SGOT: 50iu/l; Serum hydroxybutyrate dehydrogenase (HBD): 141iu/l.

RADIOLOGY & SPECIAL INVESTIGATIONS
CXR: the diaphragm appears elevated, but the lungs are clear. The heart is globular in shape. Plain abdominal film: ascites is present. Flecks of calcification are seen; Urinanalysis: no abnormality found; Paracentesis: milky fluid tinged with blood was obtained; Protein content: 31g/l (3.1g/100ml); Cytology: no malignant cells, mesothelial cells ++, monocytes ++; Gram smear: negative; Ziehl-Nielsen stain: negative.

1. List four investigations which will assist in establishing the diagnosis.

2. What is the most likely diagnosis?

CASE V

A 35-year-old policeman presented with a two week history of toothache, and a one week history of pain over the right maxilla, followed after two days by frontal headache of gradually increasing severity and exaggerated by coughing, strain and bending forwards. On the day of admission, the patient had noticed that he was dragging his right leg while getting out of bed. He was feeling shivery and seemed to be sweating excessively. The headache had become particularly acute and prolonged, brought on even by mild coughing. There was no past medical history of note, except for a blow to the right side of the head two months before, received while on duty. This had not caused any loss of consciousness and, apart from feeling dizzy for two days, he had recovered well.

On examination, he was febrile with a temperature of 37.6°C, and somewhat drowsy. Speech was normal. Pulse 80/min regular, blood pressure 130/70mmHg. Lungs and heart were normal. There was nothing of note in the abdomen. Examination of the central nervous system revealed a swollen left optic disc. There was weakness of the right leg in a pyramidal distribution, and reflexes were increased in the right leg with an extensor plantar response on that side. The rest of the neurological examination was unremarkable.

Investigations

Hb: 15.6g/dl (15.6g/100ml); MCV: 80fl (80μm^3); WBC: 10.8 × 10^9/l (10,800/mm^3); Neutrophils: 79%; Lymphocytes: 12%; ESR: 48mm/h; Sodium: 131mmol/l (131mEq/l); Potassium: 3.8mmol/l (3.8mEq/l); Bicarbonate: 23mmol/l (23mEq/l); Chloride: 93mmol/l (93mEq/l); Urea: 3.8mmol/l (23mg/100ml); Liver function tests: normal; Blood sugar: 5.7mmol/l (103mg/100ml); Urinanalysis: normal; CXR: normal.

1. What are the three most important investigations that should be carried out at this stage?

2. What is the most likely diagnosis?

Data Interpretations

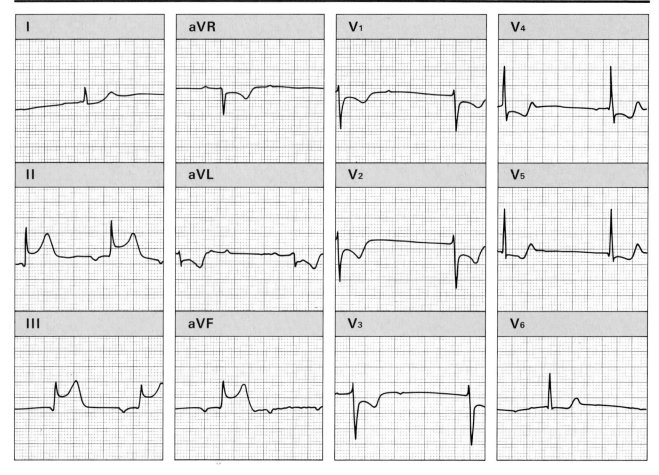

1. List three abnormalities in this ECG.

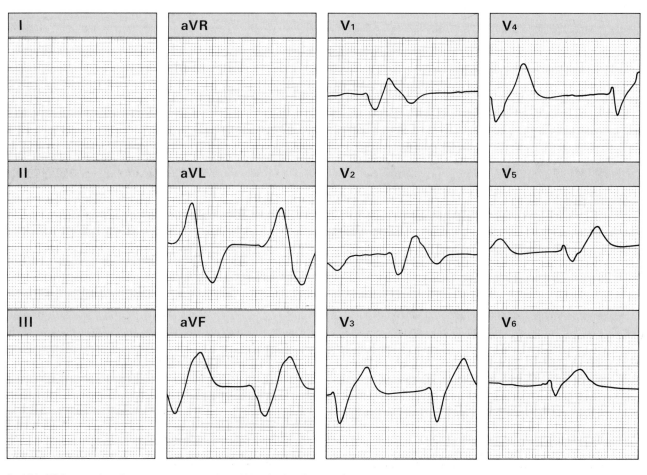

2. This ECG was taken from a comatose patient. What is the diagnosis?

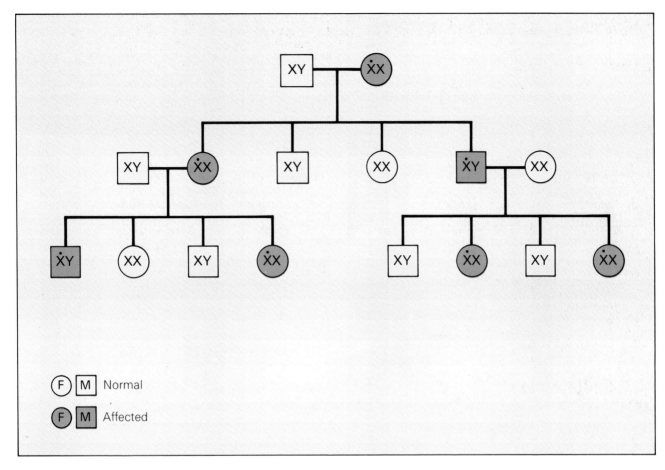

(F) (M) Normal

(F) (M) Affected

3. **(a)** What mode of inheritance is demonstrated?
   (b) List one condition which follows this mode of inheritance.

4. A 36-year-old woman is admitted for treatment of predominantly right heart failure.
   Vital capacity: 2.0l; FEV$_1$: 1.6l; Transfer factor: low; Residual volume: 1.1l.
   (a) What pulmonary defect is present?
   (b) Suggest two investigations which would elucidate its aetiology.

5. A 14-year-old boy noticed over the course of a week several small bruises on his arms and legs. Ten days before he had suffered from a coryzal illness. On the day of admission, there had been a severe epistaxis and haemorrhagic bullae were found in his mouth.
   Hb: 11.3g/dl (11.3g/100ml); Platelets: 9 × 10^9/l (9,000/mm^3); Blood film otherwise normal.
   (a) What is the presumptive diagnosis?
   (b) List two diagnostically useful investigations.

6. A 9-year-old girl is admitted with a short history of tiredness and recent bruising.
   Hb: 8.6g/dl (8.6g/dl); PCV: 0.31 (31%); MCV: 84fl (84μm^3); Reticulocytes: 0.3%; Platelets: 32 × 10^9/l (32,000/mm^3); WBC: 5.6 × 10^9/l (5,600/mm^3); Neutrophils: 13%; Lymphocytes: 41%; Lymphoblasts: 12%.
   (a) What is the diagnosis?
   (b) List two essential investigations.

7. A 45-year-old businessman gives a 15 month history of frequent attacks of central abdominal pain and occasional loose motions.
   Hb: 13.1g/dl (13.1g/100ml); MCV: 102fl (102μm^3); γGT: 115U/l; Faecal fat: 73mmol/24 hours on a 100gm fat diet.
   (a) Suggest two possible diagnoses.

(b) List three investigations which would assist the diagnosis.

8. An 85-year-old man is receiving treatment for chronic visual failure.
   Sodium: 141mmol/l (141mEq/l); Potassium: 3.1mmol/l (3.1mEq/l); Bicarbonate: 3.8mmol/l (3.8mEq/l); Chloride: 125mmol/l (125mEq/l); PaCO$_2$: 1.94kPa (14.5mmHg); pH: 7.04.
   Suggest a possible cause of this metabolic derangement.

9. A 24-year-old woman is investigated for nocturia. On examination, she is found to be hypertensive (165/100mmHg).
   Sodium: 142mmol/l (142mEq/l); Potassium: 3.9mmol/l (3.9mEq/l); Bicarbonate: 23mmol/l (23mEq/l); Urea: 4.6mmol/l (28mg/100ml).
   Following a two-litre 0.9% saline infusion over four hours, her electrolytes are as follows:
   Sodium: 148mmol/l (148mEq/l); Potassium: 3.1mmol/l (3.1mEq/l); Bicarbonate: 28mmol/l (28mEq/l).
   (a) Suggest two diagnostically useful investigations.
   (b) What is the most likely diagnosis?

10. A 63-year-old man undergoes an oral 75g glucose tolerance test as part of his investigations for weight loss.

Time (min)	Blood Glucose (mmol/l)
0	4.8
30	13.6
45	7.8
60	4.7
90	3.8
120	4.2

   (a) What abnormality is shown?
   (b) List four possible causes.

Answers

1. Gas in the biliary tree ★★★★
   Barium in the biliary tree ★★★★
   The patient had had a sphincterotomy. Gas in the biliary tree can also be due to: the passage of a gallstone; surgical anastomoses, e.g. choledocho-jejunostomy; perforated duodenal ulcer into the common bile duct; trauma.

2. Crohn's disease of the small intestine ★★★★
   Coeliac disease 0
   Terminal ileitis 0
   The characteristic X-ray finding is segmental involvement of the bowel, most often the terminal ileum, the segments of involved ileum being separated from each other by 'skip areas' of normal mucosa. Narrowing of the lumen, the so-called 'string sign of Kantor', represents a functionally contracted irritable segment or, at a later stage of the disease, fibrotic stenosis. Proximal pre-stenotic dilatation of the small bowel is present.

3. (a) Erythema marginatum ★★★★
   (b) Rheumatic fever ★★★★
       Still's disease ★★★★
   Erythema marginatum (or circinatum) of the skin is the characteristic cutaneous manifestation of acute rheumatic fever, occurring in 10–20% of childhood cases. It comes and goes, it is a multiform type of erythema, and consists of roughly circular lesions seen in the extremities, the trunk and occasionally the face, that spread centrifugally leaving a clear centre. The erythema blanches on pressure; the lesions tend to coalesce so that, although individual areas are iris-like, the larger areas are serpiginous in outline.

4. (a) Papilloedema ★★★★
       Papillitis 0
       Central retinal vein occlusion 0
       Central retinal artery occlusion 0
   (b) Raised intracranial pressure ★★★★
       Malignant hypertension ★★★★
       Raised CSF protein, e.g. Guillain-Barre syndrome ★★★★
       Hypoparathyroidism ★★
       Hypercapnia ★★

5. Conn's adenoma ★★★★
   Phaeochromocytoma 0
   The 'canary yellow' cut surface of the tumour is characteristic of an aldosterone-secreting adenoma. This is in contrast to the greyish haemorrhagic tumour seen with phaeochromocytomas.

6. Argyrosis ★★★★
   Wilson's disease ★
   Onycholysis 0

7. Left atrial myxoma ★★★★
   intracardiac tumour ★★★★
   Myxomas arise as pedunculated tumours extending through the walls of the cardiac chamber. They are considered to be true neoplasms.

8. Acute lymphoblastic leukaemia ★★★★
   Leukaemia ★★
   Infectious mononucleosis 0
   The lymphoblasts show a high nuclear cytoplasmic ratio, and the nucleus may be cleft. Often, one or two nucleoli may be present. About 28% of acute lymphoblastic leukaemia are of T cell, and 5% of B cell origin. The rest are 'null' cells.

9. Retinoblastoma ★★★★
   Cataract 0
   There is loss of the red reflex in the left eye. A convergent strabismus is present.

10. Hypernephroma ★★★★
    Renal tuberculosis 0
    Hydronephrosis 0
    Polycystic kidneys 0
    The IVU shows a left upper pelvic mass which is compressing the calyces The appearances are those of a hypernephroma.

11. Infectious mononucleosis ★★★★
    Streptococcal pharyngitis ★★★★
    Diphtheria ★★★★
    Candidiasis ★★

12. (a) Fusiform swelling of m.i.p. joints of the left hand ★★★★
    (b) Still's disease ★★★★
        Juvenile rheumatoid arthritis ★★★★
    Clinical features of Still's disease include high fever, transient morbilliform rash, leucocytosis, uveitis and a low frequency of rheumatoid factor (10%), and subcutaneous nodules. Both monoarticular and polyarticular forms may occur.

13. Hypercalcaemia ★★★★
    Hypercholesterolaemia 0
    Calcium crystals have been deposited around the limbus of the eye. Causes include:
    Primary hyperparathyroidism;
    Tertiary hyperparathyroidism;
    Sarcoidosis.

14. Low grade haemolytic anaemia ★★★★
    Cholelithiasis ★★★★
    Leg ulcers 0
    Aplastic crises 0
    The elliptical cells are those of hereditary elliptocytosis. In those patients who manifest haemolysis, the spleen is the specific site of sequestration and destruction, and splenectomy induces long term remission. Only 10% of affected individuals manifest significant shortening of the red cells.

15. Mycosis fungoides ★★★★
    Cutaneous lymphoma ★★★★
    Psoriasis ★
    Eczematous dermatitis 0
    Drug eruption 0
    This is a primary cutaneous T cell lymphoma. The lesions are indurated and plaque-like, with scaling and erythema. Histologically, Pautrier s microabscesses, atypical cells are nested within the epidermis; an infiltrate of atypical mononuclear cells and larger hyperchromatic cells ('mycosis cells') are present.

16. Intestinal obstruction ★★★★
    Intussusception ★★★★
    Volvulus ★★★★
    Appendicitis ★★★★
    Anaphylaxis (in sensitised host upon death of worm) ★★★★
    Obstruction of biliary tree ★★★★
    Pneumonitis ★★
    This is the nematode *Ascaris lumbricoides*. The female (20–35cm) is larger than the male (15–30cm) which often has a curly tail. On ingestion of infective eggs by man, the larvae hatch in the small intestine and penetrate its wall whence they are carried by the blood and lymphatic system to the lungs. This stage is often associated with fever, cough and haemoptysis, and a high blood eosinophilia. The larvae then migrate (like hookworm and strongyloides) up the respiratory passages and into the oesophagus.

17. Tuberculous ulceration ★★★★
    Small bowel ulceration ★
    Salmonellosis 0
    The long axis of the ulcers is characteristically transverse around the bowel. The undermined edges of the ulcers are also typical. These lesions are associated with bleeding and a tendency to perforation and fistula formation.

18. Empyema necessitans ★★★★
    Infected sebaceous cyst 0

19. Variegate porphyria ★★★★
    Porphyria cutanea tarda ★★
    Acute intermittent porphyria 0
    Pemphigoid 0
    Cutaneous symptoms of variegate porphyria include dermal abrasion, superficial erosions and blister formation after trivial trauma. Excessive mechanical fragility is confined to exposed parts of the skin. Light exposure is an important pathogenic factor. Hyperpigmentation and hypertrichosis may occur. These symptoms may occur alone, or together with acute transient attacks of abdominal pain and neuropathy. Biochemically large amounts of copro and protoporphyrin are present in the bile and faeces.

20. Frontal meningioma ★★★★
    Subdural haematoma 0
    Glioma 0
    The uniform raised density and contrast enhancement of the lesion (almost bony) is characteristic. Meningiomas are in general ovoid and well circumscribed. The external carotid artery generally supplies the tumour, whereas on the internal carotid angiogram the vessels are seen to be displaced.

ANSWERS TO CASE HISTORIES

Case I

1. Serum 17 α-hydroxyprogesterone ★★★★
   24h urinary pregnanetriol ★★★★
   9a.m. plasma ACTH estimation ★★★★
   24h urinary ketosteroids ★★
   9a.m. testosterone ★★
   9a.m. DHEAS ★★
   9a.m. androstenedione ★★

2. Congenital adrenal hyperplasia ★★★★
   21-hydroxylase deficiency ★★★★
   Adrenal virilising tumour ★
   There is no evidence of salt wasting. The findings are suggestive of CAH due to 21-hydroxylase deficiency. This is the commonest form of CAH, affecting one in 100,000 of the population. Cortisol synthesis is blocked at the 17α-hydroxyprogesterone → 11 deoxycortisol step.

Case II

1. CSF examination ★★★★
   EEG ★★★★
   Blood cultures ★★★★
   Thiamine level ★★★★
   Blood glucose ★★★★
   Blood and urinanalysis for drugs ★★
   Prothrombin time ★

2. Wernicke's encephalopathy ★★★★
   Hepatic porto–systemic encephalopathy ★★★★
   Series of seizures complicating alcoholism ★★★★
   Subdural haematoma ★★★★
   Central pontine myelinolysis ★★
   The EEG examination would be useful for excluding the triphasic waves of hepatic failure or epileptiform discharges. This patient had developed Wernicke's encephalopathy as a result of recurrent vomiting from his pyloric stenosis. Early objective signs of the disease include bilateral weakness or paralysis of the lateral conjugate gaze. Horizontal nystagmus is almost always present, as is vertical nystagmus particularly on upward gaze. Rarely, ptosis complete paralysis of eye movements, miosis and

unreactive pupils are present. Unsteadiness of gait is invariable.

Case III

1. Blood film ★★★★
   Bone marrow aspirate ★★★★
   Measurement of glycosyl ceramide-β-glycosidase activity ★★★★
   Antinuclear factor/double-stranded DNA antibodies ★★
   Acid phosphatase level ★★
   Haemoglobin electrophoresis 0

2. Gaucher's disease ★★★★
   Lymphoma ★★
   Leukaemia ★
   Slipped epiphysis 0
   Legg-Perthes disease 0
   Gaucher's disease (glycosyl ceramide lipidosis) is characterised by abnormal accumulation of glucocerebrosides in reticulo-endothelial cells, secondary to deficiency of an enzyme which degrades glycolipids. The increasing mass of storage cells accounts for most of the clinical manifestations – hepatomegaly, lymph node enlargement and bone lesions. The chronic non-neuronopathic adult form of the disease is the most common. The morphological hallmark of Gaucher's disease is the Gaucher cell, a round or polyhedral pale reticulum cell 20–80μm in diameter with a small eccentrically placed nucleus and a wrinkled crumpled silk cytoplasm. It is best seen from a bone marrow aspirate.

Case IV

1. Laparoscopy and biopsy ★★★★
   Culture of peritoneal fluid for tubercle ★★★★
   CT scan of abdomen (to detect lymph nodes etc.) ★★★★
   Ultrasound of abdomen ★★★★
   Liver biopsy ★★
   Mantoux test ★★
   Needle biopsy of parietal peritoneum (Abrams needle) ★★

2. Peritoneal tuberculosis ★★★★
   Disseminated malignancy ★★
   Peritoneal involvement may be the sole manifestation of tuberculosis.
   The most frequent clinical presentation is of relatively abrupt onset of unexplained ascites.

Case V

1. Sinus X-rays ★★★★
   CT scan of the head with enhancement ★★★★
   Blood cultures ★★★★
   Angiogram ★★★★
   LP if CT scan normal ★★

2. Subdural abscess ★★★★
   Left frontal lobe abscess ★★
   Cerebral thrombophlebitis ★★

ANSWERS TO DATA INTERPRETATIONS

1. Acute inferior myocardial infarction (M.I.) ★★★★
   Acute M.I. with reciprocal changes in V_1–V_5 ★★★★
   Complete heart block ★★★★

2. Hyperkalaemia ★★★★
   The ECG changes of hyperkalaemia begin with the development of tall tent shaped T waves, decreased amplitude of P waves, and later by atrial asystole. Intraventricular block with widening of the QRS complex leads to the development of a sine wave pattern, and ultimately to ventricular standstill. Changes in the ECG are seen initially with [K^+] of 7mmol/l with cardiac standstill

Answers

occurring at 10mmol/l. The changes shown can be immediately reversed by intravenous calcium lactate (2g).

3. **(a)** Dominant X-linked trait ★★★★
   (b) Vitamin D resistant rickets ★★★★
   Xgᵃ erythrocyte antigen ★★★★

The X chromosome bearing the affected gene is designated by a small dot.

4. **(a)** Restrictive lung defect ★★★★
   Obstructive lung defect 0
   (b) Rheumatoid factor ★★★★
   Kveim test ★★★★
   Transbronchial/open lung biopsy ★★★★
   Antinuclear factor ★★★★
   Chest radiograph ★★
   Anti-centromere antibody ★★

5. **(a)** Idiopathic thrombocytopenic purpura ★★★★
   Autoimmune thrombocytopenia ★★★★
   Post-viral thrombocytopenia ★★
   (b) Bone marrow aspirate ★★★★
   Anti-platelet antibody estimation ★★★★

A bone marrow aspirate will demonstrate marked hyperplasia of megakaryocytes, consistent with peripheral destruction of platelets. A number of *in vitro* test systems are available to demonstrate platelet antibodies in ITP. Treatment of ITP is with prednisolone 1–2mg/kg during the period of maximal thrombocytopenia. In 80% of patients the disease is self-limiting.

6. **(a)** Acute lymphoblastic leukaemia ★★★★
   Leukaemia ★★
   Infectious mononucleosis 0
   (b) Bone marrow examination ★★★★
   Cytochemical tests on blasts ★★★★
   Cell membrane phenotyping, to look for common ALL
      antigen ★★★★
   Cytogenetics ★

7. **(a)** Chronic pancreatitis with malabsorption ★★★★
   Pancreatic malabsorption secondary to alcoholism ★★★★
   Coeliac disease ★★
   Giardiasis ★
   (b) Plain abdominal X-ray to demonstrate pancreatic
      calcification ★★★★
   Lundh test ★★★★
   ERCP (endoscopic retrograde cholangio-
      pancreatography) ★★★★
   Pancreatic CT scan ★★
   Jejunal biopsy ★★
   Inspection of stools for cysts/ova ★★

8. Hyperchloraemic acidosis induced by carbonic anhydrase
      inhibitors (e.g. acetazolamide, mafenamide) ★★★★
   Metabolic acidosis ★★
   Chronic renal failure ★
   Lactic acidosis 0
   The anion gap $(Na^+ + K^+) - (HCO_3 + Cl^-)$ is $(141 + 3.1) - (125 + 3.8) = 15.3mmol/l$, which is normal; this excludes an acidosis caused by some other species such as lactic acid or ketoacids.

9. **(a)** Plasma renin ★★★★
   Aldosterone ★★★★
   CT scan of the adrenals ★★
   Iodocholesterol scan of the adrenals ★★
   Venous catheterisation for aldosterone ★★
   (b) Primary hyperaldosteronism ★★★★
   Mineralocorticoid-related hypertension ★★
   Essential hypertension 0

The saline provocation test suggests that excess mineralo-corticoid is present, as hypokalaemia has been induced.

10. **(a)** Lag storage curve ★★★★
    (b) Thyrotoxicosis ★★★★
    Severe liver disease ★★★★
    Reactive hypoglycaemia (normal variant) ★★★★
    Reactive hypoglycaemia following gastrectomy or
       gastrojejunostomy ★★★★
    Diabetes mellitus 0

Paper 5

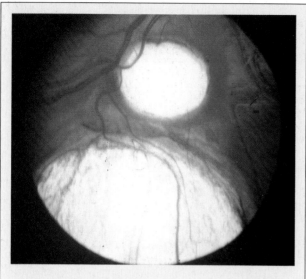

1. What is the diagnosis?

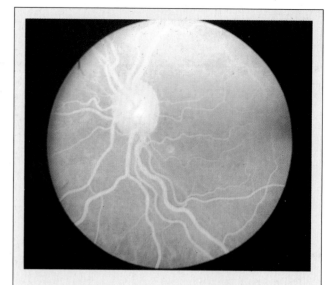

2. What abnormality is shown?

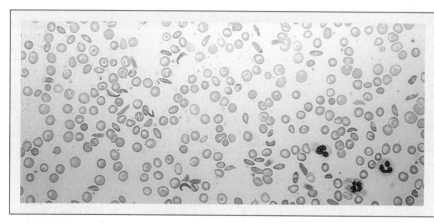

3. What is the diagnosis?

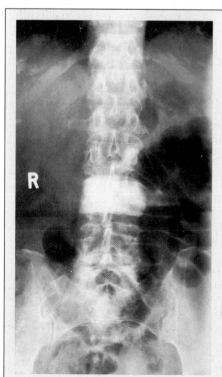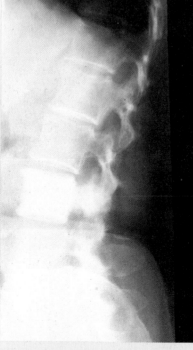

4. These films of the lumbar spine were from a 65-year-old woman undergoing investigations for back pain.
What is the most likely cause for the abnormality shown?

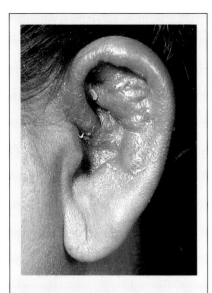

5. What is the likely cause of this lesion which appeared intermittently?

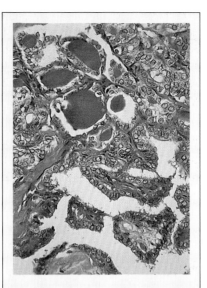

6. This is the histology from a thyroid nodule. What is the diagnosis?

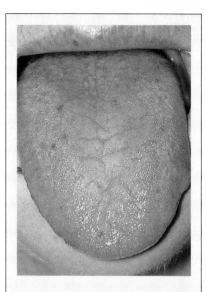

7. List two pulmonary complications of this condition.

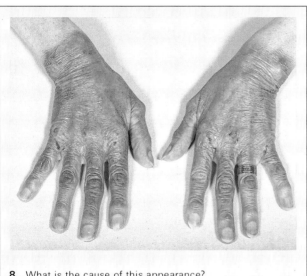

8. What is the cause of this appearance?

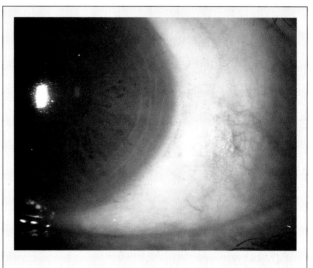

9. What is the diagnosis?

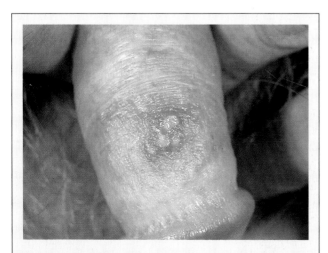

10. This lesion appeared seven days after sexual exposure. What is the likely diagnosis?

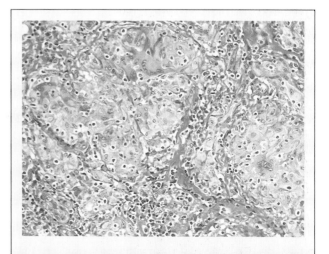

11. This section was from a lymph node biopsy. What is the most likely diagnosis?

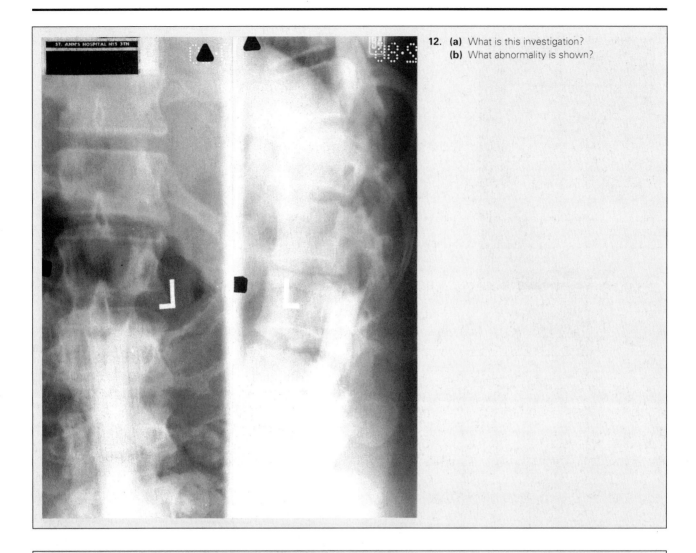

12. **(a)** What is this investigation?
    (b) What abnormality is shown?

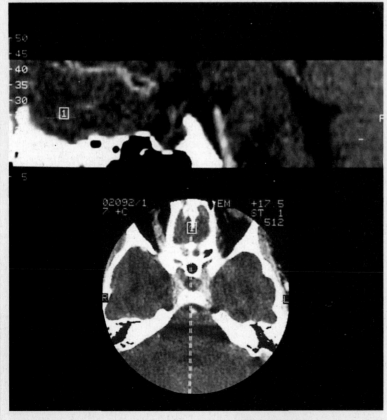

13. This investigation was carried out in a 26-year-old woman with galactorrhea and amenorrhea.
    (a) What investigation is shown?
    (b) What abnormality is present?

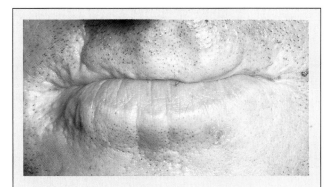

14. What is the likely diagnosis of this appearance?

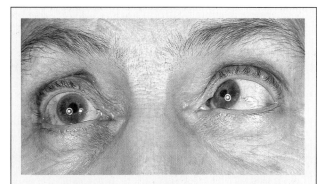

15. This patient is attempting to look up and to the right. What is the diagnosis?

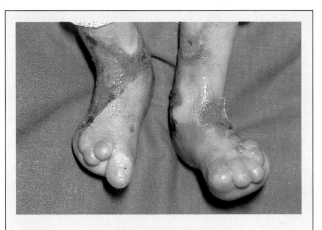

16. What is the likely cause of this skin condition?

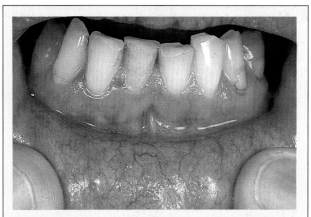

17. These are the gums of a man under investigation for weight loss, diarrhoea, and abnormal liver function tests. What is the likely diagnosis?

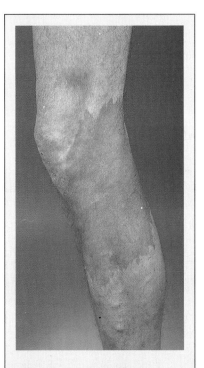

18. What is the diagnosis?

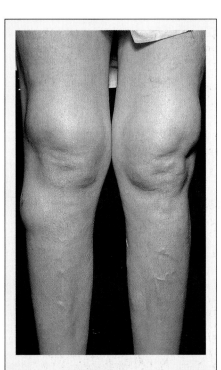

19. What is the likely cause of this appearance?

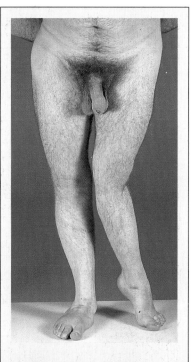

20. This man had similar deformities in his upper limbs.
(a) What is the diagnosis?
(b) List two complications of this condition.

CASE I

A 61-year-old West Indian woman was admitted for investigation of poorly controlled hypertension. Her hypertension had been diagnosed twenty-five years before, and since that time she had been prescribed a variety of agents to control her blood pressure, but because of poor compliance, this was never brought under control. Recently, the patient had suffered several episodes of giddiness brought on by exertion, and often postural. There had been no history of palpitations, exertional dyspnoea or angina. For a number of years, she had suffered from nocturia two to three times at night, as well as from occasional headaches.

On examination, she was obese and weighed 84kg. Pulse 60/min regular, blood pressure 230/130mmHg supine and 160/100mmHg standing. A small goitre was noted. The cardiac apex was laterally displaced about 3cm, and the jugulovenous pulse was not raised. The apex was of a thrusting quality, and auscultation revealed a grade 2/6 ejection systolic murmur, best heard at the apex, with no radiation. The lungs were clear, and in the abdomen 1cm of liver was palpable. Fundal examination revealed arterial narrowing and some AV nipping. The rest of her physical examination was unremarkable.

Investigations

Hb: 14.6g/dl (14.6g/100ml); WBC: 6.9 × 10⁹/l (6,900/mm³); ESR: 13mm/h; Sodium: 144mmol/l (144mEq/l); Potassium: 2.8mmol/l (2.8mEq/l); Bicarbonate: 28mmol/l (28mEq/l); Creatinine: 0.14mmol/l: Liver function tests: normal; Spot urinary sodium concentration: 26mmol/l(26mEq/l); Spot urinary potassium concentration: 47mmol/l (47mEq/l); CXR: heart moderately enlarged with a prominent left ventricular border; ECG: sinus rhythm, evidence of left ventricular hypertrophy and strain.

1. List three investigations which would assist in this patient's management.

2. List two possible diagnoses.

CASE II

A 27-year-old woman was admitted to hospital following onset of a convulsive episode. Ten weeks previously, she had given birth to her first child. This had been an unplanned pregnancy, and she was suffering a rather severe postnatal depression. She had had one episode of depression in late adolescence which had required hospitalisation. Because of her inability to sleep at night, she was prescribed sleeping tablets and diazepam for day-time sedation. Four days after starting this medication, she began to complain of generalised pain and drowsiness. Her husband noted her to be confused. She also began to complain of severe central abdominal pain, not associated with any change in bowel habit. On the day prior to admission, she suddenly felt light-headed in the bathroom, and fell striking her head. The following morning, while in bed, she had a grandmal seizure, and was admitted.

On examination, she was drowsy with evidence of mild weakness of the right side. There was no neck stiffness. Her temperature was 38.4°C, pulse 140/min, blood pressure 170/120mmHg. There was no hepatosplenomegaly, but the abdomen was tender. Pelvic examination was normal. There was weakness of dorsiflexion of the right wrist, and diplopia on lateral gaze. Fundal examination was normal.

Investigations

Hb: 12.6g/dl (12.6g/100ml); WBC: 16.4 × 10⁹/l (16,400/mm³); Neutrophils: 80%; ESR: 28mm/h; Sodium: 138mmol/l (138mEq/l); Potassium: 4.6mmol/l (4.6mEq/l); Bicarbonate: 24mmol/l (24mEq/l); Chloride: 103mmol/l (103mEq/l); Creatinine: 120μmol/l (1.36mg/100ml); Urea: 5.6mmol/l (2mg/100ml); Liver function tests: normal; Blood glucose: 5.8mmol/l (104mg/100ml); VDRL TPHA: negative; Urinanalysis: normal; CXR: mild enlargement of the cardiac silhouette; ECG: normal.

1. List three investigations which would help in establishing the correct diagnosis.

2. Give a likely cause for this patient's acute presentation.

CASE III

A 34-year-old school teacher was admitted to hospital in a state of confusion. The history given by his wife was that for two days he had been unwell and pyrexial. On the day before admission, he had become somewhat confused, uttering unintelligible words, with disorientation in time and place. On that evening, he had attempted to write a letter but found that he was writing incoherently. In his past medical history he had been well, but for the last three years he had been taking small doses of benzo-diazepine to control anxiety.

On examination, there was no neck stiffness, but temperature was 38.6°C. His memory function appeared particularly poor. Pulse 110/min regular, blood pressure 120/90mmHg. Examination of the heart and lungs was normal, and abdominal examination was unremarkable. The fundi appeared normal. Examination of the remainder of the central nervous system revealed no focal abnormality.

Investigations

Hb: 14.2g/dl (14.2g/100ml); WBC: 6.4 × 10⁹/l (6,400/mm³); ESR: 47mm/h; Urea and electrolytes: normal; Liver function tests: normal; Blood sugar level: 6.2mmol/l (110mg/100ml); CXR: normal; Urinanalysis: normal; CSF cells: 65 × 10⁹/l (65,000/mm³); Lymphocytes: 95%; Red cells: 12/mm³; Glucose: 4.6mmol/l (81mg/100ml); Protein: 0.8g/l (80mg/100ml).

1. List three essential investigations in the patient's management.

2. What is the most likely diagnosis?

CASE IV

A 68-year-old woman was admitted to hospital following the abrupt onset on severe tinnitus, vertigo, nausea, vomiting and dysarthria. Her symptoms had started about six hours before admission. In her medical history she had been hypertensive, and was on regular medication with a thiazide diuretic. In addition, she had been treated monthly with vitamin B12 injections for a macrocytic anaemia discovered when she was 55 years old. The only family history of note was that a sister had become demented at the age of 71 and had required long-term institutionalised care.

On examination, she was somewhat distressed with a pulse of 96/min irregular, and a blood pressure of 165/100mmHg. A soft, apical systolic murmur was audible at the base of the heart. She was alert and well orientated in place and time, but nystagmus was elicited with a fast component maximal on gaze to the left. Abduction of the left eye was limited, and a left lower motor neurone facial weakness was noted. The patient was moderately dysarthric, and examination of the limbs showed her to be ataxic in the left arm and leg. She was unable to sit unsupported.

Otherwise, muscle tone, power and sensory testing were normal. Reflexes were slightly brisker on the right side, and the plantar reflexes were flexor. Her symptoms gradually improved over the following 72 hours, but shortly thereafter she once again became obtunded with no change in focal signs. She began to complain of headache and became incontinent on the ward. She was given 4mg dexamethasone every four hours, but after 24 hours her conscious level deteriorated.

1. List two investigations which would assist in the patient's management.

2. What was the most likely diagnosis when she was first admitted?

3. Suggest a possible explanation for her deterioration.

CASE V

A 26-year-old saleswoman was admitted to hospital as an emergency, complaining of severe pain in the right hypochondrium, of acute onset. The pain was worse on breathing, and had become associated with nausea and some vomiting. Her general health had been good in the past except that, six weeks before, she had noticed a vaginal discharge which was not offensive. Her regular boyfriend was being treated with a tetracycline preparation for recent dysuria and clear penile discharge. As a child, she had suffered from rheumatic fever but was not known to have any complication of this illness. Her mother had died at the age of 60 from breast cancer, and her father drank heavily. Her general health had otherwise been good.

On examination, she was pyrexial at 37.4°C and not icteric. There was tenderness in the right hypochondrium, but no evidence of hepato- or splenomegaly. A rub was audible over the liver. Bowel sounds were normal. Pelvic examination revealed some tenderness on cervical excitation; a greyish vaginal discharge was present.

Examination of the central nervous system, the heart and lungs was normal. Pulse 70/min regular, blood pressure 120/80mmHg. Her pain remained constant and severe for eight days, confined to the right hypochondrial region. It gradually subsided over the following few days without specific treatment.

Investigations

HAEMATOLOGY

Hb: 13.1g/dl (13.1g/100ml); WBC: 6.4×10^9/l (6,400/mm³); Normal differential count.

BIOCHEMISTRY & SPECIAL INVESTIGATIONS

Sodium: 136mmol/l (136mEq/l); Potassium: 4.2mmol/l (4.2mEq/l); Bicarbonate: 25mmol/l (25mEq/l); Chloride: 102mmol/l (102mEq/l); Urea: 4.7mmol/l (2mg/100ml); Creatinine: 80μmol/l (0.09mg/100ml); Bilirubin: 9μmol/l (0.5mg/100ml); Alkaline phosphatase: 86iu/l (1.2KAU/100ml); Total protein: 68g/l (6.8g/100ml); Albumin: 37g/l (3.7g/100ml); Calcium: 2.4mmol/l (9.4mg/100ml); phosphate: 0.88mmol/l (3.2mg/100ml); Serum glutamic oxaloacetic transaminase (SGOT): 51iu/l; Serum amylase activity: 212 Somogyi units; Glucose: 4.6mmol/l (83mg/100ml); VDRL TPHA: negative.

RADIOLOGY

CXR: normal; Oral cholecystogram: normal; Barium meal: no ulcers seen.

1. Suggest two investigations which would help in the patient's management.

2. Suggest a likely diagnosis.

Data Interpretations

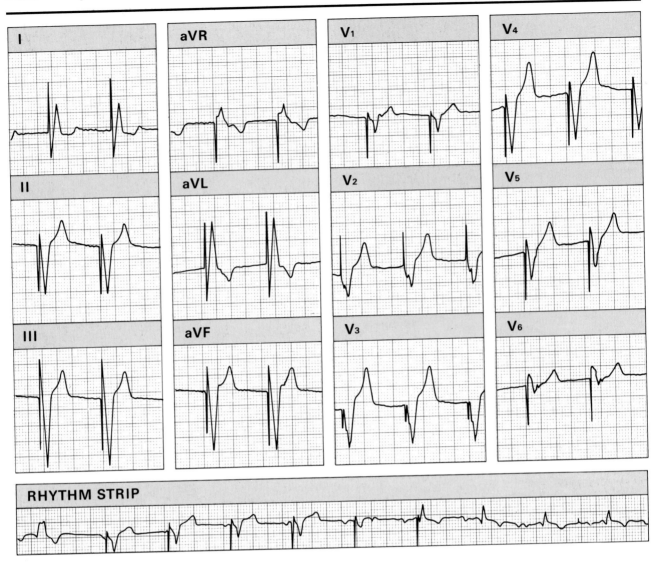

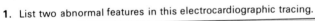

1. List two abnormal features in this electrocardiographic tracing.

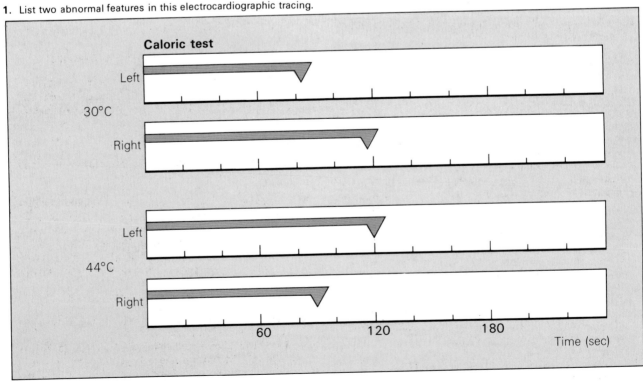

2. What conclusion can be reached from this caloric test?

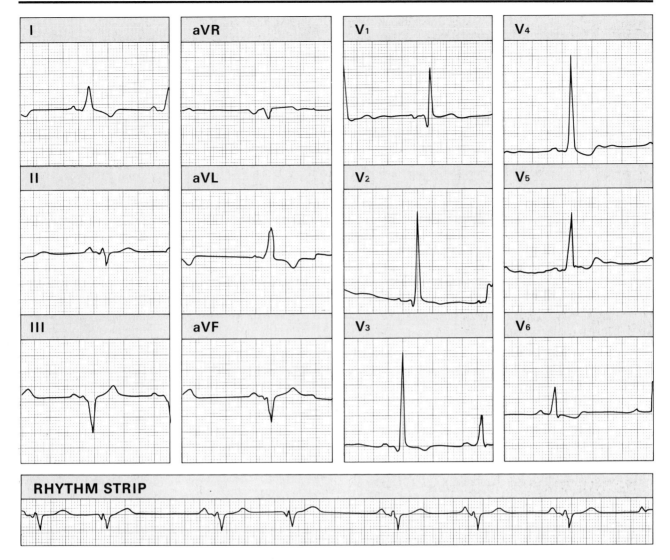

| I | aVR | V₁ | V₄ |
| aVR | | | |

RHYTHM STRIP

3. What abnormalities are present on this ECG?

4. A 54-year-old bachelor businessman was investigated for dysarthria and progressive inability to recall recent events. CSF examination: Pressure: $135 mmH_2O$; Cells: $58 \times 10^9/l$ ($58,000/mm^3$); Lymphocytes: 98%; Protein: 1.5g/l (150mg/100ml).
   (a) Give two diagnostically useful investigations.
   (b) Suggest a likely diagnosis.

5. A 25-year-old school teacher complains of palpitations and episodes of feeling faint. A 24 hour urinary VMA estimation was $39\mu mol$ (normal range: $10-35\mu mol$/24 hours). A pentolinium test (2.5mg iv) is carried out.

Time (min)	Noradrenaline (nmol/l)	Adrenaline (nmol/l)
0	2.40	0.88
10	1.02	0.18

What inferences can be drawn from the above results?

6. An 85-year-old woman was admitted with severe lower sternal pain lasting about six hours. 24 hours later, the following results were obtained.
   Bilirubin: $17\mu mol/l$ (1mg/100ml); Alkaline phosphatase: 259iu/l (thermolabile); Total protein: 68g/l (6.8g/100ml); Albumin: 37g/l (3.7g/100ml); SGOT: 87iu/l; HBD: 290iu/l.
   Suggest two likely underlying diagnoses.

7. A 68-year-old man is investigated because of severe bruising after apparently minimal trauma.
   PT: 12 sec (control 12 sec); PTTK: 35 sec (control 36 sec); Platelets: 225,000/mm³; Hess test: strongly positive.

Suggest four possible causes.

8. A 35-year-old woman is investigated for weight gain, irregular menstruation and lethargy.
   Hb: 17.3g/dl (173g/100ml); PCV: 0.55 (55%); Potassium: 2.8mmol/l (2.8mEq/l); Bicarbonate: 31mmol/l (31mEq/l);

OGTT (75g)	Time (min)	Glucose (mmol/l)
	0	5.1
	30	16.4
	120	12.8

   (a) List three diagnostically useful investigations.
   (b) What is the probable diagnosis?

9. A 16-year-old boy undergoes a xylose absorption test as part of an investigation for possible cystic fibrosis. After an overnight fast, he takes 5mg orally and collects his urine for the subsequent five hours into two bottles.
   Total excreted over five hours: 1.25g; Percentage excreted over first two hours: 38%; Percentage over following three hours: 62%.
   What inferences can be drawn from these results?

10. A 61-year-old coal miner gives a ten year history of progressive breathlessness.
    FEV_1: 0.8l/sec (predicted 2.44-3.30); FVC: 2.1 l (predicted 3.28-4.43); Residual volume: 5.1l (predicted 1.76-2.38); KCO: 0.37mmol/min/kPa/l (predicted 1.35-1.83); Insp. R_{AW}: 0.29 (<0.2).
    What is the likely underlying abnormality?

Answers

ANSWERS TO SLIDE INTERPRETATIONS

1. Coloboma of the eye ★★★★
   Choroidoretinitis 0
   Colobomas are developmental defects that arise from imperfect closure of the fetal cleft, and show in consequence an absence of any or all of the structures which lie along the corresponding lower nasal or temporal sectors of the eye. They are usually bilateral and may be complete, extending from the pupil to the optic nerve, with a corresponding indentation of the lens. Here, the coloboma is incomplete involving localised oval patches of the fundus partitioned by tongues of normal tissue.

2. Lipaemia retinalis ★★★★
   This is caused by fat-laden blood, appearing as cream in both retinal arteries and veins. It may be seen in uncontrolled diabetes mellitus and in hypertriglyceridaemias.

3. Sickle cell anaemia (Hb$\alpha_2 \beta^{s}_2$) ★★★★
   Iron deficiency anaemia 0
   Leucoerythroblastic anaemia 0
   Darkly staining sickle and target cells are seen in the blood film, and there is a nucleated red cell. In HbS there is a variable degree of anaemia (Hb 6–9g/dl), an elevated reticulocyte count, anisochromia and poikilocytosis. As a child with HbS gets older, the haematological changes of hyposplenism develop, with the appearance of Howell-Jolly bodies. An elevated reticulocyte count is always present. Sickling may be easily provoked in the laboratory by taking a drop of blood and mixing it with a drop of freshly prepared sodium metabisulphite.

4. Secondary deposit from breast carcinoma (post DXR or chemotherapy) ★★★★
   Secondary deposit from pelvic tumour ★★★★
   Metastasis from colonic neoplasm ★★★★
   Lymphomatous deposit from Hodgkin s disease ★★★★
   Carcinoid deposit ★★
   There is a sclerotic lesion in the body of L3, involving the pedicles as well as the pedicles of L2. The two common causes of sclerotic bone lesions are metastases from breast in a female and prostate in a male. Lymphoma may cause a single sclerotic vertebral body. Lack of expansion of the vertebra makes this unlikely to be Paget's disease of bone.

5. Relapsing polychondritis of the ear ★★★★
   Cellulitis of the ear ★★
   Allergic skin reaction ★
   This is an intermittently progressive disease marked by inflammatory destruction of cartilage. Cartilage of the external and inner ears, larynx, trachea, bronchi and nose may be involved. The replacement of cartilage by fibrous tissue will eventually lead to the development of laryngeal and tracheal stenosis. Pyrexia, anaemia and a raised ESR are common. Joint cartilage, the sclera, and the aortic valve ring may also be involved.

6. Papillary carcinoma of the thyroid ★★★★
   Follicular carcinoma of the thyroid 0
   The section shows a typical mixture of neoplastic papillae and neo-plastic colloid-containing follicles. The nuclei are crowded, irregular in shape, and empty looking. The papillae of these tumours consist of elongated branching fibrovascular cores covered by a single layer of epithelium. The follicles contain eosinophilic colloid, or appear empty. In approximately 60% of the tumours, the nuclei of both papillae and follicles are characteristically empty-looking with a prominent rim due to linear condensation of chromatin against the nuclear membrane. These nuclei are described as having a ground glass appearance, and they are large, misshapen and overlapping. Approximately 50% of these tumours contain scattered small spherical laminated calcified bodies called psammona bodies or calspherocytes.

7. Haemoptysis ★★★★
   Pulmonary arteriovenous fistulae ★★★★
   Pulmonary haemorrhage ★★
   This is Rendu-Osler-Weber syndrome (hereditary haemorrhagic telangiectasia), an autosomally dominant inherited condition which usually becomes clinically manifest after puberty. The characteristic lesion is thin-walled and sac-like, formed of vascular cells, that blanches with pressure. Lesions occur in the mouth, stomach, elsewhere in the gut and in the lungs. Iron deficiency anaemia can be a long-term complication.

8. Pellagra ★★★★
   Niacin deficiency ★★★★
   Contact dermatitis ★
   Kwashiorkor 0
   Pellagra dermatosis is characteristical symmetrical and occurs on the sun-exposed parts of the body. Erythema is followed by chronic hypertrophy, with thickened scaly skin which is hyperkeratinised and pigmented. Pressure points are affected, and Casal s necklace is pathognomonic. The tongue is usually scarlet and painful. Diarrhoea and dementia are common. Pellagra may occur secondary to malabsorption in diarrhoeal and liver diseases, and in alcoholism. It may complicate prolonged isoniazid therapy, carcinoid syndrome, and Hartnup disease.

9. Bitot's spot ★★★★
   Vitamin A deficiency ★★★★
   Pinguecula 0
   With advanced Vitamin A deficiency, dryness (xerosis) of the conjunctiva occurs, affecting the exposed parts; this results from defective mucin production and keratinisation of the epithelial cells. The cornea may be affected by a punctate keratopathy which proceeds to liquefaction and dissolution of the corneal substance (keratomalacia). With advanced deficiency a panoph-thalmitis resulting in phthisis bulbi or corneal ectasia may occur.

10. Herpes genitalis ★★★★
    Syphilitic chancre 0
    Scabies 0
    Behçet's syndrome 0
    Both HSV1 and HSV2 can cause genital herpes. Following a primary infection, the virus persists in the presacral ganglia in a latent form, and may be reactivated. Factors precipitating recurrences include immunosuppression, corticosteroids, inter-current infection, menstruation in females and stress or fatigue.

11. Sarcoidosis ★★★★
    Non-caseating granuloma ★★★★
    The fully formed granuloma of sarcoidosis consists of a sharply demarcated collection of epithelioid cells with a variable, usually small number of lymphocytes around it. Multinucleate giant cells may contain crystalline and conchoidal bodies. Hyaline fibrosis usually replaces the granulomas if they do not resolve.

12. (a) A water soluble myelogram ★★★★
        Myelogram ★★
    (b) Complete obstruction at the level of L1/2 ★★★★

13. (a) Contrast-enhanced CT scan of the pituitary fossa with sagittal reconstruction ★★★★
        CT scan of pituitary fossa ★★
    (b) Lucent area in the base of the pituitary fossa ★★★★
        Pituitary microadenoma ★★★★

14. Syphilitic rhagades around the mouth ★★★★
    Scleroderma ★
    Hypogonadism 0
    This is a cutaneous stigma of late congenital syphilis. Other stigmata include gummas, periostitis, interstitial keratitis, synovitis (Clutton's joints), neurolabyrinthitis, Hutchinson's teeth, saddle nose, high arched palate, and Parrot's nodes on the skull.

Optic atrophy and choroiditis may also occur.

15. Right abducent nerve palsy ★★★★
This may occur in:
Diabetes mellitus;
Raised intracranial pressure (false localising sign);
Wernicke's encephalopathy;
Any cause of mononeuritis multiplex.

16. Epidermolysis bullosa dystrophica ★★★★
Epidermolysis bullosa ★★.
Severe burns 0
This can be transmitted by dominant and recessive autosomal inheritance. The onset is at birth; its course is often severe with deformity and can be fatal. Even normal looking skin has an abnormal texture and blisters easily. Repetitive blistering leads to fusion of the fingers and toes, and gross scarring and dystrophy of the nails. Mucosal involvement of the mouth and oesophagus can lead to oesophageal stenosis. The disorder is thought to be secondary to a collagen defect in the dermis.

17. Addison's disease ★★★★
Haemochromotosis ★
There is gingival pigmentation, best seen between the teeth. Abnormal liver function tests are not uncommon in untreated Addison's disease, and are usually manifested by elevated liver enzymes. The diagnosis of Addison's can be confirmed with a short synacthen test, which will show a flat cortisol response. A long synacthen test (1mg s/c) may be performed also. This will likewise be flat in primary renal insufficiency, whereas there is a delayed rise in cortisol in secondary renal failure.

18. Neurofibromatosis ★★★★
Tuberose sclerosis ★
Café-au-lait spots have been reported in association with pulmonary stenosis and temporal dysrhythmia, with no other signs of neurofibromatosis in either case. Four types of lesions are pathognomonic of tuberose sclerosis: (a) Firm, discrete, yellowish or telangiectatic papules around the nasolabial furrow, cheeks and chin – 'adenoma sebaceum of Pringle'; (b) The shagreen patch; (c) Ovoid or linear leaf-shaped, white macules on the trunk or limbs; (d) Periungal fibromata (Koenen's tumours).

19. Rheumatoid arthritis ★★★★
Bilateral knee joint effusions ★★★★
There is gross synovial thickening, bilateral knee effusions and some wasting of the quadriceps muscle.

20. (a) Osteogenesis imperfecta tarda ★★★★
Rickets ★
(b) Otosclerosis ★★★★
Growth stunting ★★★★
Scoliosis deformity ★★★★
Fractures ★★★★
In osteogenesis imperfecta tarda, fractures are often subperiosteal, causing no pain or tenderness, hence they are allowed to heal with deformity. They unite readily, with the callus usually more dense than in normal bone. Other features include blue sclerae.

ANSWERS TO CASE HISTORIES

Case I

1. Serum aldosterone estimation ★★★★
Plasma renin estimation ★★★★
CAT scan of adrenals ★★★★
Iodocholesterol scan after dexamethasone suppression ★★★★
Captopril suppression test ★★

Adrenal venous catheterisation for aldosterone levels ★★
Creatinine clearance ★★
Urinary vanillyl mandelic acid/metanephrine estimation ★
Intravenous urogram ★

2. Conn's adenoma ★★★★
Nodular hyperplasia of adrenals ★★★★
Essential hypertension with previous diuretics ★★★★
Liquorice addiction ★★
Cushing's syndrome ★★
Phaeochromocytoma 0
Several features in this case indicate the need to exclude primary hyperaldosteronism: hypokalaemic alkalosis, mild hypernatraemia, hyperkaliuria, postural hypotension and refractory hypertension. An elevated serum aldosterone in the presence of a low renin level suggests primary hyperaldosteronism. Glucose intolerance may also occur. The consumption of carbenoxolone sodium in liquorice addiction may cause hypokalaemic alkalosis. Rarer causes include renin-secreting tumours (haemangioperi-cytoma) and congenital adrenal hyperplasia. The differential diagnosis between a Conn's adenoma (CA) and nodular hyperplasia (NH) may be aided by: (a) The aldosterone response to a graded angiotensin II infusion – a large aldosterone increment is seen in NH but a flat response with CA; (b) Serum aldosterone taken after overnight supine rest (8a.m.) and after remaining erect for four hours. A falling aldosterone suggests CA, and no change or an increased aldosterone suggests NH.

Case II
1. Schwartz-Watson test ★★★★
Electroencephalography ★★★★
CT scan of head ★★★★
Lumbar puncture ★★★★
Blood cultures ★★★★
Spirometry ★★

2. Acute intermittent porphyria (AIP) ★★★★
Acute encephalomyelitis ★★
Cerebral abscess ★
Benzodiazepine intoxication 0
AIP is inherited as a dominant trait; it is associated with recurrent attacks of abdominal pain, gastrointestinal dysfunction and neurological complications. Attacks are rarely seen before the third or fourth decade, and are characterised by episodes of colicky abdominal pain usually in the context of the soft abdomen. Leucocytosis, fever, lack of bowel sounds, gastric dilatation, motor peripheral neuropathy (varying from mild weakness in one limb to complete flaccid paraplegia), with absent deep tendon reflexes, ophthalmoplegia, optic atrophy, facial palsy and dysphagia are all recognised complications. Functional/emotional disturbances frequently precede the acute episode. Sinus tachycardia has been ascribed to vagal neuropathy. Attacks may be precipitated by barbiturates, sulphonamides, griseofulvin and oestrogens, all of which are metabolised by hepatic microsomal enzymes. Characteristically, there is excessive urinary δ aminolaevulinic acid and porphobilinogen.

Case III
1. CAT scan of brain ★★★★
Blood cultures ★★★★
CSF culture ★★★★
Electroencephalogram ★★★★
Magnetic resonance imaging of brain ★★
Herpes simplex virus serology ★★
Brain biopsy ★★

2. Herpes simplex encephalitis ★★★★
Cerebral abscess ★★★★
Viral encephalitis ★★

Case IV
1. Contrast enhanced CAT scan of brain ★★★★

Echocardiography ★★★★
Blood cultures ★★★★
Electrocardiogram ★★★★

2. Brainstem or cerebellar infarction secondary to embolus ★★★★
Brainstem encephalitis ★★★★
Brainstem haemorrhage ★★★★
Basilar artery thrombosis ★★

3. Brainstem/cerebellar oedema in wake of infarct or
haemorrhage ★★★★
Hydrocephalus in wake of cerebellar infarction ★★★★
Progression of basilar artery thrombosis ★★

Case V

1. Cervical swab for microscopy and culture ★★★★
Chlamydial serology ★★★★
Ventilation-perfusion lung scan ★★★★
Blood cultures ★★★★
Urine culture and microscopy ★★★★
Liver ultrasound ★★

2. Chlamydial perihepatitis ★★★★
Ruptured hepatic adenoma ★★
Pleurisy ★★
Chlamydial salpingitis ★★
Liver abscess ★★
Gonococcal perihepatitis ★★
Acute cholecystitis ★
Pyelonephritis ★
Gonococcal or chlamydial perihepatitis (Fitz-Hugh-Curtis syndrome)
is caused by ultra-abdominal spread of the infection to the right
upper quadrant. Adnexal tenderness is usually present on pelvic
examination. There is shoulder pain and a friction rub over the liver
may be heard – these are not found in uncomplicated acute
cholecystitis. Other generalised complications include endocarditis
and a febrile illness presenting as a 'pyrexia of unknown origin'.

ANSWERS TO DATA INTERPRETATIONS

1. Ventricular demand pacemaker ★★★★
1° HB (First degree heart block) ★★★★
Incomplete right bundle branch block ★★★★

2. Left directional preponderance ★★★★
Any other answer 0
The two stimuli that would usually produce nystagmus to the left
fail to do so (i.e. cold in the left ear and warm in the right ear);
this shows that the nerve endings are normal, but that the brainstem mechanism that controls gaze to the left is defective.

3. Bigeminus rhythm ★★★★
Left axis deviation ★★★★
Left atrial hypertrophy ★★★★
Left bundle branch block ★★★★
Incomplete right bundle branch block ★★★★

4. (a) Serum syphilis serology ★★★★
CSF, VDRL, TPHA ★★★★
CSF gamma globulin level ★
Lange colloidal gold curve ★
(b) Parenchymatous neurosyphilis ★★★★
Neurosarcoid ★
Viral encephalitis ★
Frontal lobe tumour 0
Alzheimer's disease 0
Multiple sclerosis 0
Four main types of acquired neurosyphilis are recognised:
Meningovascular: It occurs within twelve years of primary

infection and affects meninges and meningeal vessels. It may
present as a CVA, isolated cranial nerve palsies or papillitis. A
chronic leptomeningitis is present with Huebner's endarteritis
obliterans. Fever is usually absent.
Parenchymatous: The meninges become thickened and
opacified, and ventricular walls become studded with ependymal
granulations. Gross gyral and convolutional atrophy occurs.
Clinically, intellectual impairment, hyperactive reflexes with
extensor plantar reflexes and Argyll Robertson pupils are found.
Tremor of the hands and 'trombone' tongue occur.
Tabes dorsalis: It is characterised by lightning pains in the limbs,
ataxia and sphincter disturbance, high stepping gait, failing
vision, diplopia, neurogenic arthropathy and perforating ulcers.
Asymptomatic: Diagnosed on CSF examination; pleocytosis
(mainly lymphocytes) and a raised protein are usually found.

5. Normal response ★★★★
Phaeochromocytoma present 0
The ganglion blocking drug pentolinium, when given
intravenously in a dose of 2.5mg will, in normal subjects,
suppress circulating noradrenaline and adrenaline into the normal
range. In autonomous catecholamine-secreting tumours, there is
failure of suppression.

6. Myocardial infarction ★★★★
Paget's disease of bone ★★★★
Thermolabile alkaline phosphatase is of bony origin, and Paget's
disease is the most likely underlying cause.

7. Scurvy ★★★★
Amyloidosis ★★★★
Cushing's syndrome ★★★★
Qualitative platelet defect ★★★★
The findings suggest bleeding due to a vascular defect. Other
causes include drug-induced purpura, senile purpura, Henoch-
Schönlein purpura, dysproteinaemias, Ehlers-Danlos syndrome
and pseudoxanthoma elasticum. Of the genetically determined
platelet disorders, Bernard-Soulier syndrome (functionally
defective giant platelets) and storage pool disease may cause
extensive bruising and purpura.

8. (a) Circadian rhythm study for cortisol ★★★★
Dexamethasone suppression test ★★★★
Insulin tolerance test ★★★★
Urinary-free cortisol ★★★★
ACTH level ★★★★
CT scan of adrenals ★★★★
Chest and skull X-ray ★★★★
(b) Cushing's syndrome ★★★★
Primary hyperaldosteronism ★★
Hypokalaemic alkalosis, a diabetic glucose tolerance test and
polycythaemia should suggest glucocorticoid excess (Cushing's
syndrome), especially caused by ectopic ACTH secretion.

9. Mild malabsorption ★★★★
Although the total five hour absorption is within the normal range
(>23%), 50% or more of this should occur within the first two
hours. The results are compatible with mild malabsorption. D-
xylose is an inert pentose which is absorbed by the small intestine
and excreted entirely by the kidney, having passed unchanged
through the liver. False positive results are not uncommon, and
may be related to age, renal disease, delayed gastric emptying,
hypothyroidism and xylose-induced osmotic diarrhoea.

10. Emphysema ★★★★
Severe airflow limitation with trapping ★★★★
Asthma ★
Emphysema is a condition that, strictly, can only be diagnosed
histologically. The inspiratory resistance is quite low, and the rise
in RV with the reduced KCO suggests that the surface for
gaseous exchange is abnormally reduced. In asthma, a raised
KCO would be expected.

Paper 6

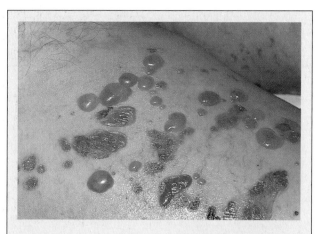

1. This is the thigh of a 65-year-old woman. She had complained of pruritic erythematous lesions prior to this eruption.
   What is the diagnosis?

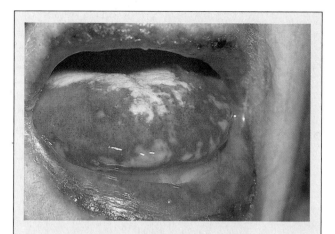

2. The trunk of this patient was covered with vesicobullous and urticarial lesions.
   What is the diagnosis?

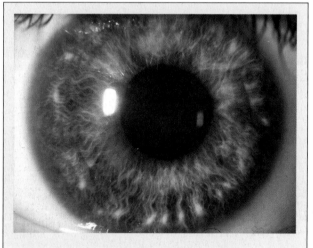

3. This is the eye of a 17-year-old girl with mental retardation.
   What is the diagnosis?

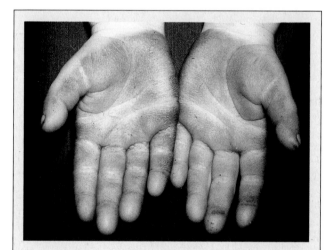

4. (a) What is the diagnosis?
   (b) List one recognised association.

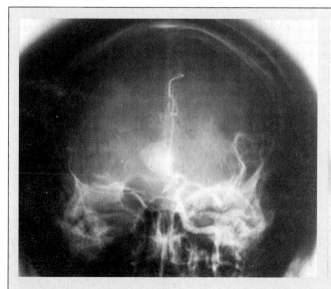
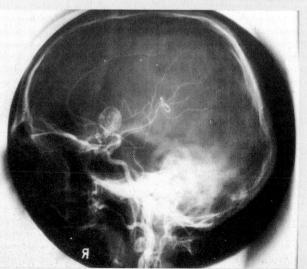

5. What abnormality is shown?

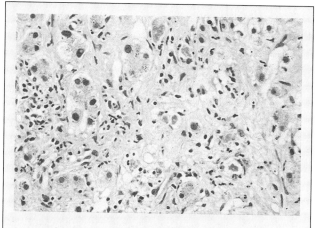

6. This is a section of a liver biopsy from a 55-year-old man with chronic liver disease.
What is the underlying cause?

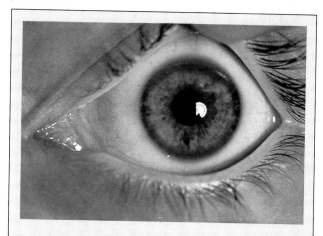

7. What is the diagnosis?

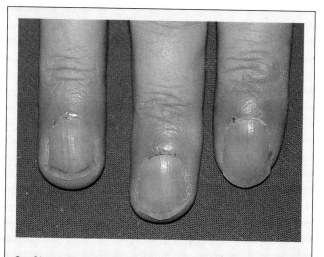

8. Give three possible causes for the appearance shown.

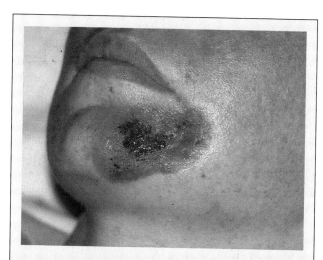

9. What is the diagnosis?

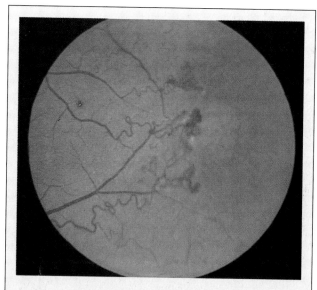

10. What is the diagnosis?

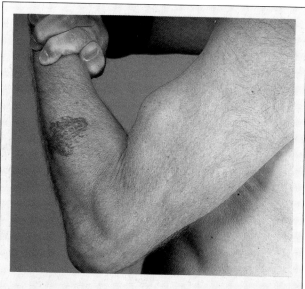

11. What physical sign is demonstrated?

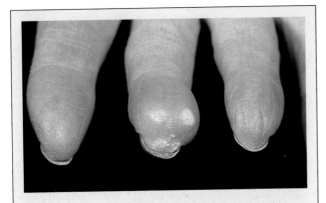

12. (a) What is the likely cause of this appearance?
    (b) Suggest an alternative diagnosis.

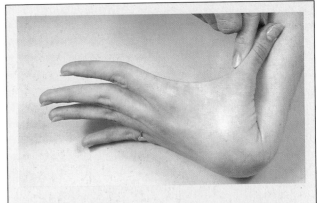

13. List three conditions which may be associated with this physical sign.

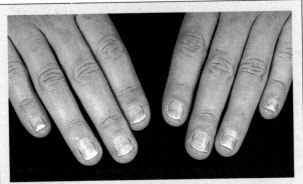

14. These are the fingers of a 38-year-old woman under treatment for weight loss and atrial fibrillation. What physical sign is shown?

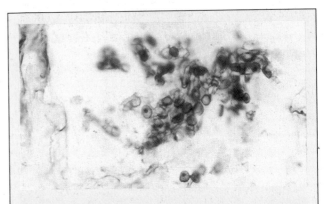

15. This is a methenamine silver stain of a lung biopsy. What is the diagnosis?

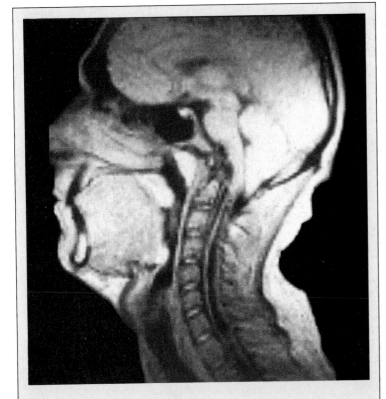

16. This man was investigated for spasticity in the lower limbs. What is the diagnosis?

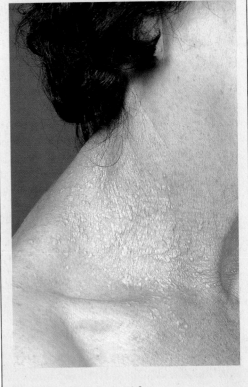

17. What is the diagnosis?

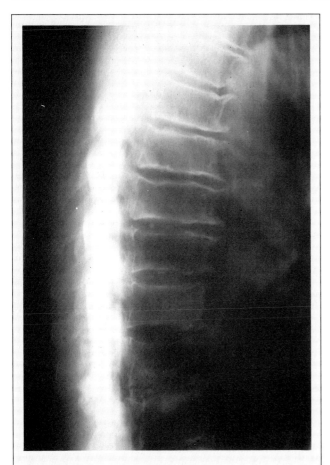

18. What is the cause of this radiological appearance?

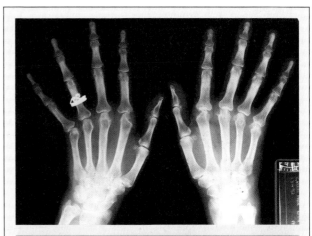

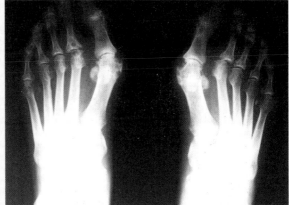

19. These are the hands and feet of a 50-year-old female. List three abnormalities apparent in these radiographs.

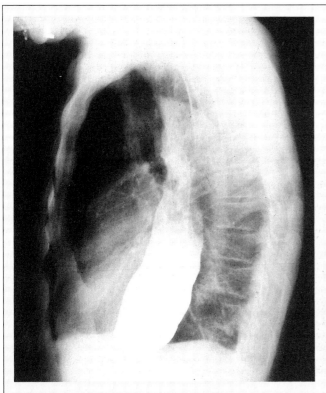

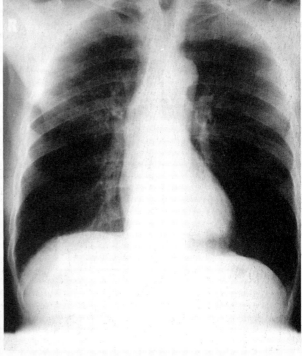

20. These views of the oesophagus were taken during a barium swallow. Symptoms of dysphagia had been progressing over the past 10 years. **(a)** What abnormalities are shown?
(b) What is the likely diagnosis?

Case Histories

CASE I

A 54-year-old man was admitted as an emergency complaining of shortness of breath which had come on over the preceding 24 hours. A week before, he had woken up at night with severe dyspnoea, relieved only on standing. On the day of admission he had experienced two to three small haemoptyses, and had developed low back pain radiating downwards in the left leg, associated with cold feet. In his medical history, five years before he had undergone a mitral valve replacement with a Starr Edwards prosthesis for rheumatic heart disease. Lately, the patient had been taking diuretics, digoxin and an anticoagulant.

On examination, he was grey and cold, and very dyspnoeic at rest. Pulse 100/min irregular, blood pressure 110/65mmHg. The jugulovenous pressure was raised to 6cm. Pitting oedema was present. In the chest there were fine crepitations from the mid zones. Examination of the pulses revealed absence of the femoral pulses. Auscultation of the heart revealed absence of the prosthetic mitral first sound. There were no other murmurs.

Investigations

HAEMATOLOGY
Hb: 11.2g/dl (11.2g/100ml); MCV: 94fl (94μm^3); WBC: 10.8 × 10^9/l (10,800/mm^3); Platelets: 250 × 10^9/l (250,000/mm^3); Blood film: polychromasia present; ESR: 12mm/h.

BIOCHEMISTRY
Bilirubin: 22μmol/l (1.3mg/100ml); Alkaline phosphatase: 65iu/l (8KAU/100ml); Serum glutamic oxaloacetic transaminase (SGOT): 28iu/l; Albumin: 34g/l (3.4g/100ml); Urinanalysis: urobilinogen ++; no bile present.

1. List three investigations which would be diagnostically useful.

2. What two complications are likely to have occurred?

CASE II

A 47-year-old teacher was admitted for investigation of swelling of the right orbit and of the right side of the face. She had been in good health in the past, but three months before she first noticed that her right eye was itching and discharging. Over the ensuing weeks the right orbit gradually swelled, became reddened and then violaceous in colour, with a decreasing right palpable fissure. Her GP initially treated her with chloramphenicol eye drops to no avail. One month before admission, the swelling seemed to spread to the right side of the face, and the patient began to complain of pain over the right maxilla. Two weeks before admission she developed a light yellow, non-offensive, nasal discharge. This occurred through the night and often stained her pillow by morning. Her general health had been good in the past, apart from an appendicectomy at the age of 19. She had never married and had had regular periods until six months before, when they had become slightly heavier and less regular. She was on no medication, and there was no family history of note.

On examination, she was a pleasant, well-orientated lady, who was pyrexial with a temperature of 37.6°C. Pulse 70/min regular, blood pressure 130/90mmHg. Her jugulovenous pulse was not raised. There was no lymphadenopathy, and examination of heart and lungs was entirely normal. The abdomen was normal, as was pelvic examination. There was a slight orbital swelling on the right which was indurated and violaceous in colour, and minimally tender. The right eye-ball was proptosed. The swelling of the right maxilla was very tender to palpation. Examination of the anterior nares revealed crusting of the nasal septum and a small perforation at the apex of the nose. When the right eyelid was retracted, it was clear that the patient was unable to elevate her right eye fully, and was developing diplopia in upward as well as lower gaze.

Investigations

HAEMATOLOGY
Hb: 11.9g/dl (11.9g/100ml); MCV: 84fl (84μm^3); WBC: 6.8 × 10^9/l (6,800/mm^3); Normal differential count; ESR: 74mm/h; Platelets: 470 × 10^9/l (470,000/mm^3).

BIOCHEMISTRY & RADIOLOGY
Urea: 4.4mmol/l (27mg/100ml); Sodium: 139mmol/l (139mEq/l); Potassium: 3.8mmol/l (3.8mEq/l); Chloride: 98mmol/l (98mEq/l); Bicarbonate: 24mmol/l (24mEq/l); Bilirubin: 16μmol/l (0.97mg/100ml); Alkaline phosphatase: 98iu/l (13KAU/100ml); Total protein: 78g/l (7.8g/100ml); Albumin: 37g/l (3.7g/100ml); Calcium: 2.45mmol/l (9.6mg/100ml); PO$_4$: 0.98mmol/l (3.14mEq/l); SGOT: 37iu/l; ECG: normal; Skull X-ray: there is an opacification of the right maxillary sinus, with no other abnormalities seen; Urinanalysis: normal; Mantoux test: negative at 1/1000.

1. Suggest three investigations which might assist in the diagnosis.

2. Suggest two possible diagnoses.

CASE III

A 46-year-old businessman consulted his GP because of a two week history of drenching night sweats and headache. He was known to be a mild essential hypertensive, but had otherwise been in good health. His blood pressure was usually well controlled on a thiazide diuretic alone. Recently, he had found it difficult to concentrate at work, but this would only last half a day and subsequently he would return to normal. He drank one third of a bottle of wine and smoked ten cigarettes a day. There was no family history of note. He was referred to Outpatients, where further questioning revealed that his symptoms had started since returning from a Mediterranean cruise four weeks before. In addition to the night sweats, he complained of extreme fatigue and of occasional pain in his joints and muscles. There was accompanying anorexia, and he had lost approximately 3kg in weight since the onset of his illness. Just before his outpatient consultation, he developed some redness of his right eye, and complained of an excessive number of 'floaters'.

On examination he looked unwell, with a temperature of 37.6°C. Pulse 86/min regular, blood pressure 120/70mmHg. Cardiac auscultation revealed an ejection systolic murmur best heard at the apex. Lungs were clear. Some shotty lymph nodes were palpable in the axillae and groins. In the abdomen, the liver was enlarged by 3cm and smooth, but the spleen was not palpable. Rectal and central nervous system examinations were normal.

HAEMATOLOGY

Hb: 12.8g/l (12.8g/100ml); MCV: 83fl (83μm³); WBC: 6.6 × 10⁹/l (6,600/mm³); Neutrophils: 1.9 × 10⁹/l (1,900/mm³); Platelets: 244 × 10⁹/l (244,000/mm³); ESR: 14mm/h.

BIOCHEMISTRY

Urea: 5.2mmol/l (32mg/100ml); Creatinine: 0.08mmol/l (0.9mg/100ml); Sodium: 139mmol/l (139mEq/l); Potassium: 4.2mmol/l (4.2mEq/l); Bicarbonate: 26mmol/l (26mEq/l); Chloride: 98mmol/l (98mEq/l); Bilirubin: 20μmol/l (1.3mg/100ml); Alkaline phosphatase: 146iu/l (18.9KAU/100ml); Total protein: 74g/l (7.4g/100ml); Albumin: 42 g/l (4.2g/100ml); Calcium: 2.5mmol/l (9.8mg/100ml); Phosphate: 1.2mmol/l (4.43mg/100ml); SGOT: 47iu/l; Serum hydroxybutyrate dehydrogenase: 94iu/l; VDRL TPHA: negative; Urinalysis: normal.

RADIOLOGY & SPECIAL INVESTIGATIONS

CXR: bilateral hilar lymphadenopathy noted; a small effusion on the right; Ophthalmic examination: inflammatory cells present in the anterior chamber; Flare +; Intraocular pressure: 23mmHg.

1. List five investigations which would assist in establishing a diagnosis.

2. List two possible diagnoses.

CASE IV

A 6-year-old girl was brought to Casualty by her mother because of progressive recent onset of unsteadiness of gait. The child had been well until six days before, when, after attending a birthday party, she had developed profuse diarrhoea and vomiting. This had continued over 24 hours, necessitating a visit by the GP who prescribed an antiemetic. Despite this, the child continued to vomit, and it was only after intramuscular administration of antiemetics that her symptoms settled down. Her GP encouraged oral fluid intake and thought about admitting the child to hospital, particularly as she was very dehydrated.

With the easing of her symptoms, the parents decided to manage the child at home. As her gastrointestinal symptoms subsided, the child began to complain of tingling and numbness in the legs. This progressed over a number of hours, and she found that she was tripping when walking. She complained of a mild headache. Following an episode of incontinence she was admitted to hospital. There had been no fitting and no tongue biting. In her past history, she had been healthy, with normal developmental milestones and no serious illnesses of note; she had, however, been susceptible to middle ear infection, particularly after upper respiratory tract infections. The last episode was two months previously, when this had required antibiotic therapy.

On examination, the child looked unwell, and still had dry mucosal membranes and slightly sunken eyeballs. She was mildly tachypnoeic; pulse 100/min regular, blood pressure 90/70mmHg. Her chest was clear and heart normal. The abdomen was still slightly tender. On central nervous system examination the cranial nerves were normal. Tone, power and coordination reflexes in the arms appeared normal. In the legs, there was dysaesthesia to pin prick and light touch from the hips downwards, and reflexes both in the knees and ankle jerks were brisk. There were three beats of ankle clonus, on both the left and the right. The right plantar was

equivocal, and the left plantar definitely upgoing. Joint positional sense of the lower limbs appeared impaired. Fundal examination revealed swelling of the optic nerve heads.

Hb: 15.1g/dl (15.1g/100ml); WBC: 20 × 10⁹/l (20,000/mm³); Neutrophils: 75%; Urea: 8.2mmol/l (50mg/100ml); Creatinine: 0.12mmol/l (1.35mg/100ml); Sodium: 150mmol/l (150mEq/l); Potassium: 4.8mmol/l (4.8mEq/l); Bicarbonate: 25mmol/l (25mEq/l); Chloride: 119mmol/l (119mEq/l); Urinalysis: normal; CXR: normal.

1. List two investigations which would assist in her management.

2. What is the most likely diagnosis?

CASE V

A 52-year-old woman sought medical advice because of difficulty in walking. She had been well until three months before, when she began to complain of a sensation in her feet similar to walking in thick woollen socks. Progressively, she had become unsteady while walking, and particularly when standing in the dark or with her eyes shut. She complained of a vague pain in the back which seemed poorly localised. In her medical history, she had had a mastectomy twelve years before, following the discovery of a carcinoma, and had been well since then. Two years before, she had been involved in a road traffic accident from which she had suffered severe chest pain, but this was not ascribed to any bone injury.

On examination, she was a well-looking woman, with a right mastectomy scar. There was no lymphadenopathy. She was not anaemic or clubbed. Pulse 90/min regular, blood pressure 120/90mmHg. Examination of the heart and lungs was normal. In the abdomen there was no organomegaly, and pelvic examination was normal. On neurological examination, she appeared to have loss of joint positional sense in her toes, and of vibration sense below the upper part of the sternum. There was mild impairment to pinprick and light touch sensation below the knees. Anal tone was normal. Her gait was unsteady, and Romberg's sign was positive. Reflexes were brisk in the lower limb, and both plantar responses were equivocal.

Hb: 13.4g/dl (13.4g/100ml); WBC: 6.4 × 10⁹/l (6,400/mm³); Normal differential count; Platelets: 212 × 10⁹/l (212,000/mm³); ESR: 35mm/h; Urea and electrolytes: normal; Liver function test: normal; Urinalysis: normal; CXR: normal.

1. List three investigations which would assist in establishing a diagnosis.

2. Suggest two possible diagnoses.

Data Interpretations

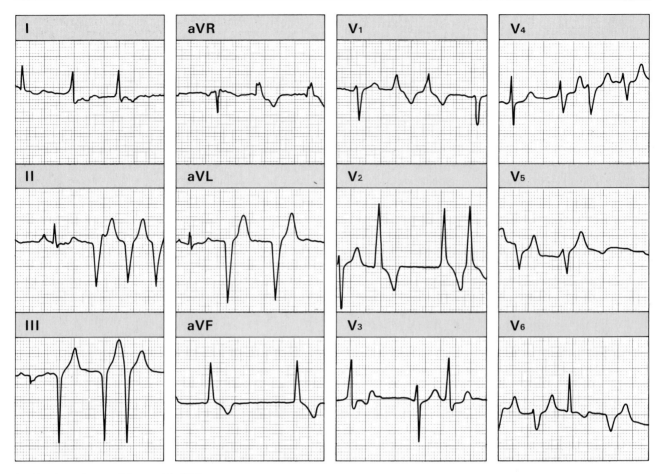

1. List three abnormalities on this ECG.

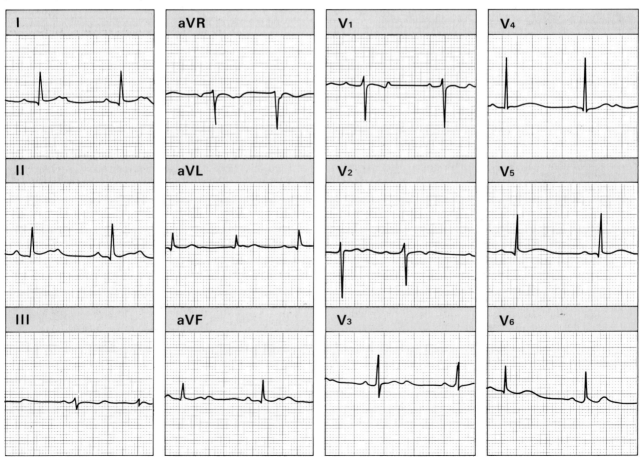

6.8 **2.** What abnormality is present on this ECG?

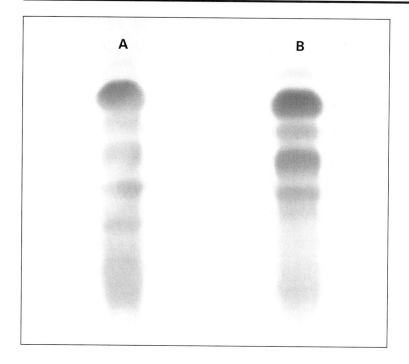

3. **A** represents the serum electrophoretic strip from a normal individual, and **B** from a patient. Suggest two possible causes for the electrophoretic appearance in **B**.

4. Two days after a sore throat, a 9-year-old girl develops gross haematuria.
   Urea: 3.6mmol/l (27mg/100ml); Sodium: 138mmol/l (138mEq/l); Potassium: 4.2mmol/l (4.2mEq/l); Creatinine clearance: 68ml/min; Urinary protein: 0.16g/24h; Urinary microscopy: red cell casts ++, granular casts ++.
   (a) What is the most likely diagnosis?
   (b) Suggest two diagnostically helpful investigations.

5. A 23-year-old girl is investigated for recent onset of secondary amenorrhoea.
   LH: 25iu/l; FSH: >50iu/l; Serum oestradiol: 105pmol/l.
   An LHRH test is carried out (100μg i.v. at time '0').

Time (min)	LH mU/l	FSH mU/l
0	24	>50
30	>50	>50
60	>50	>50

   (a) What is the likely diagnosis?
   (b) Suggest two diagnostically useful investigations.

6. A 23-year-old nurse is found unconscious. She is clinically dehydrated and hyperventilating.
   pH: 6.96; PaO₂: 17.4kPa (130.5mmHg); PaCO₂: 1.1kPa (8.25mmHg); Urea: 12.6mmol/l; Glucose: 2.1mmol/l; A urinary ferric chloride test gave a red-purple discolouration.
   (a) What is the most likely diagnosis?
   (b) Suggest two diagnostically useful investigations.

7. A 24-year-old girl was admitted to hospital following onset of jaundice. She had flu a few weeks before, and 48 hours before admission she passed dark red urine.
   Hb: 9.2g/dl (9.2g/100ml); Reticulocytes: 6%; Urobilinogen: ++; Serum bilirubin: 42μmol/l (2.5mg/100ml); Test for bilirubinuria: negative.
   (a) Suggest a possible cause for this presentation.
   (b) What is the likely cause of the discoloured urine?

8. A 36-year-old man is admitted with respiratory failure. Three minutes after receiving an intravenous drug, his respiratory function improved significantly.

Vitalograph tracing

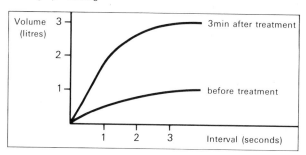

What is the most likely diagnosis?

9. A 9-year-old girl is admitted to hospital following a convulsion. Ten days before she had suffered from a diarrhoeal illness. She gave a history of recent headaches and on examination her blood pressure was 155/100mmHg.
   Hb: 8.3g/dl (8.3g/100ml); PCV: 0.26 (26%); MCV: 106fl (106/μm³); WBC: 13.7 × 10⁹/l (13,700/mm³); Platelets: 55 × 10⁹/l (55,000/mm³); Reticulocytes: 12.4%; Calcium: 1.84mmol/l (7.23mg/100ml); PO₄: 2.9mmol/l (9.3mg/100ml); Urea: 29.6mmol/l (222mg/100ml).
   (a) List three diagnostically useful investigations.
   (b) Suggest the most likely diagnosis.

10. A patient with a long-standing nephrotic syndrome develops severe pain in the left loin and haematuria.
   Sodium: 137mmol/l (137mEq/l); Potassium: 4.8mmol/l (4.8mEq/l); Bicarbonate: 20mmol/l (20mEq/l); Chloride: 98mmol/l (98mEq/l); Urea: 20mmol/l (124mg/100ml); Creatinine: 0.31mmol/l (3.5mg/100ml); Albumin: 18g/l (1.8g/100ml); Urine protein: 6.9g/24h; Urine cytology: red cells ++++.
   (a) Suggest a possible explanation for this presentation.
   (b) List two diagnostically useful investigations.

Answers

ANSWERS TO SLIDE INTERPRETATIONS

1. Bullous pemphigoid ★★★★
   Erythema multiforme ★★
   Pemphigus vulgaris 0
   Dermatitis herpetiformis 0
   Approximately 70% of patients with this condition have a serum antibody specific for the basement membrane zone of stratified squamous epithelium. The bullae are subepidermal, and acantholysis is absent in contrast to pemphigus. The eruption commonly starts with a non-specific rash on the limbs, which may be urticarial or eczematous. Bullae arise on the erythematous or normal skin; they are tense and dome-shaped, with the blisters remaining intact for several days. Corticosteroids are indicated as soon as the diagnosis is made (by histological examination). The disease runs a chronic course, and a long-term maintenance on corticosteroids is usually required.

2. Stevens-Johnson syndrome ★★★★
   (syn.: ectodermosis erosiva pluriorificialis)
   Herpetic stomatitis ★
   Drug eruption ★
   This is a severe illness of acute onset. Mouth, eyes, skin, genitalia and mucous membranes may be affected, and bronchitis and pneumonitis can occur. Initially, the oral mucous membrane shows extensive bulla formation followed by erosions, and a greyish-white membrane, so that the mouth and lips show characteristic haemorrhagic crusting. The illness can recur. The commonest association is with a preceding herpes simplex or mycoplasma pneumoniae infection. Other causes include drug sensitivity (e.g. sulphonamides), and possibly the contraceptive pill.

3. Brushfield spots ★★★★
   Down's syndrome ★★★★
   The silver-grey Brushfield spots are shown on the iris. Other ocular manifestations of Down's syndrome include hyperplasia of the iris, narrow palpebral fissures with oriental slant, frequent strabismus, epicanthus, frequent cataract and high myopia (33%).

4. (a) Tylosis ★★★★
      Diffuse palmoplantar keratoderma ★★★★
   (b) Oesophageal carcinoma ★★★★
      Darier's disease ★★★★
      Dyskeratosis congenita ★★★★
   Tylosis (Thost-Unna syndrome) is determined by an autosomal dominant gene, and is caused by an increased thickness of the horny layer. Thickening of the palms and soles is first evident in early infancy. Hyperhidrosis is frequently present, and painful fissuring is sometimes troublesome. The nails, teeth and hair are normal. Palmoplantar hyperkeratosis occurs in other syndromes, including hidrotic ectodermal dysplasia, Naegeli's syndrome, pachyonychia congenita and pityriasis rubra pilaris.

5. Anterior communicating artery aneurysm ★★★★
   Aneurysm ★
   Most intracranial aneurysms occur in a few constant situations on the circle of Willis, and most are on the anterior half of the circle. About one-third of those that rupture are on the anterior communicating or proximal anterior cerebral artery. Such aneurysms may derive their blood supply from either or both internal carotids, and are situated such that rupture may occur into either frontal lobes. Compression of local structures may produce visual field defect and hydrocephalus.

6. Alcoholic liver disease ★★★★
   Alcoholic cirrhosis ★★★★
   The cytoplasm of some of the hepatocytes contains hyaline eosinophilic clumping. These are 'Mallory bodies', which are found both in the central portion of the lobule and in close proximity to the portal scars. They are characteristic of alcoholic

hepatitis and cirrhosis. Mallory bodies may be seen in the absence of cirrhosis and have been described in primary biliary cirrhosis, non-alcoholic nutritional liver disease, hepatomas and hamartomas. Another histological hallmark of alcoholic liver disease is the giant mitochondrion.

7. Wilson's disease ★★★★
   Kayser-Fleischer rings ★★★★

8. Subacute bacterial endocarditis ★★★★
   Systemic lupus erythematosus ★★★★
   Rheumatoid arthritis ★★★★
   Polyarteritis nodosa ★★★★
   Nailfold vasculitic lesions and early clubbing are present.

9. Pyoderma gangrenosum ★★★★
   (syn.: phagedena geometrica; dermatitis gangrenosa; phagedenic pyoderma)
   Sweet's acute neutrophilic dermatosis ★
   Amoebiasis cutis ★
   Blastomycosis ★
   Causes include inflammatory bowel disease, rheumatoid arthritis, Wegener's granulomatosis, lymphoma and paraproteinaemia.

10. 'Sea fan' new vessel formation ★★★★
    Sickle cell disease with 'sea fan' neovascularisation ★★★★
    Neovascularisation ★★
    Ocular abnormalities of sickle cell disease (both SS and SC) include conjunctival changes with 'comma-shaped' capillaries, retinal changes including arterial occlusions, neovascular 'sea fan' patterns, and extensive capillary closures. Vitreous haemorrhage may be caused by bleeding neovascular membranes.

11. Ruptured biceps tendon ★★★★
    This is usually an injury of the elderly. The appearance is characteristic, as a marked ridge over the lower part of the biceps muscle when the elbow is flexed or the forearm supinated. The injury usually follows long-standing bicipital tendonitis.

12. Dermatomyositis ★★★★
    Systemic sclerosis ★★★★
    Gouty tophus ★
    Dermatomyositis is one of the causes of calcinosis cutis.

13. Ehlers-Danlos syndrome ★★★★
    Homocystinuria ★★★★
    Marfan's syndrome ★★★★
    Arthrochalasis multiplex congenita ★★★★

14. Onycholysis ★★★★
    Onychomycosis ★★
    The patient was suffering from thyrotoxicosis and the physical sign is that of Plumber's nails. The nails are frequently abnormal in thyrotoxicosis, the most common abnormality being onycholysis, where there is separation of the nail from the nail bed. Patients complain of having difficulty cleaning their nails. The condition regresses upon treatment of the hyperthyroidism.

15. Pneumocystis carinii cysts ★★★★
    Pneumonia ★
    The diagnostic feature is the presence of intra-alveolar clumps of foamy material containing the characteristic cysts which are round or oval and about 5 um in diameter. The organism may also be identified by an immunofluorescent technique. There is often associated alveolar cell hyperplasia, and interstitial invasion with lymphocytes and plasma cells. Pneumocystis pneumonia is seen in malnourished subjects, those with a background of chronic disease (e.g. Hodgkin's and leukaemia), and immuno-suppressed patients (e.g. AIDS). Treatment is with cotrimoxazole or pentamidine isethionate 4 mg/kg for 10–14 days.

16. Syringomyelia ★★★★
Multiple sclerosis 0
This MRI scan shows a syrinx in the cervical cord.

17. Pseudoxanthoma elasticum ★★★★
There has been deposition of calcium on elastic fibres. In the fully developed lesion the elastic fibres in the mid dermis are degenerate, fragmented and swollen, and mucopolysaccharide (mainly hyaluronic acid) is increased. Electron microscopically, most elastic fibres are grossly abnormal, and the early stage of elastogenesis is defective. The changes in the eyes give rise to angioid streaks. The skin lesions consist of small yellowish papules in confluent plaques often associated with telangiectasia. Obliterative arterial disease may occur.

18. Acromegaly ★★★★
Osteoporosis ★
This lateral view demonstrates new bone formation at the anterior margins of the vertebrae. The anterior edge of the intervertebral discs can be clearly identified and the vertebral bodies are increased in their anteroposterior diameter. The new bone formation is usually more marked in the dorsal than in the lumbar spine. Fistular scalloping and prominent marginal osteophyte formation are characteristic.

19. Ulnar deviation of the hands ★★★★
Valgus deformity of metacarpophalangeal, metatarso-phalangeal and middle interphalangeal joints ★★★★
Multiple marginal joint erosions ★★★★
Periarticular osteoporosis ★★★★
These are classical rheumatoid feet and hands. Early radiological changes are soft tissue swelling and periarticular osteoporosis. Later erosions of MCP, MTP and MIP joints develop with similar changes at the carpus. Ulnar deviation/valgus deformities occur. Swan neck and boutonniere deformities of the fingers may also occur.

20. (a) Smooth stricture at the oesophago-gastric junction ★★★★
Proximatal dilatation of oesophagus ★★★★
Delay in the passage of barium ★★★★
(b) Achalasia ★★★★
Scleroderma ★★
Peptic stricture ★★
Carcinoma of the oesophagus ★
The most common form of achalasia is idiopathic. Other forms include Chagas' disease, endemic in certain parts of the world, and secondary achalasia, due to carcinomatous infiltration of the myenteric plexus. Systemic sclerosis and peptic stricture are other diagnoses to consider, but the oesophagus is usually less dilated.

ANSWERS TO CASE HISTORIES

Case I

1. Echocardiogram to visualise the prosthetic mitral valve ★★★★
Doppler studies of peripheral arteries ★★★★
Prothrombin time ★★★★
Blood cultures ★★★★
Electrocardiogram ★

2. Saddle embolus to aortic bifurcation ★★★★
Thrombus formation of the mitral valve prosthesis ★★★★
Pulmonary oedema ★★★★
Subacute bacterial endocarditis ★★
Pulmonary embolus ★

Case II

1. Nasal septal biopsy ★★★★
X-ray of chest ★★★★
Biopsy of eyelid ★★★★
CT scan of orbits and sinuses ★★★★

Slit lamp examination of the eye ★★★★
Lung function tests ★★

2. Wegener's granulomatosis ★★★★
Polyarteritis nodosa ★★★★
Vasculitis ★★
Sarcoidosis ★★
This was a case of Wegener's granulomatosis. A characteristic early lesion consists of a persisting crusting, haemorrhagic granuloma of the nostril, nasal mucosa, pharynx, larynx and trachea. Involvement of the lungs and kidneys is frequent. Chest radiographs may reveal pulmonary infiltration (usually bilateral) in the lower lung, which cavitates. The necrotising arteritis can affect the kidney, causing a focal or diffuse glomerulonephritis.

Case III

1. Blood cultures ★★★★
Bone marrow culture ★★★★
Serum agglutination test for brucella ★★★★
HIV antibody titre ★★★★
ANF ★★
Liver biopsy ★★
Mantoux test ★★
Kveim test ★★
Bronchoscopy and lung biopsy ★

2. Acute brucellosis ★★★★
Sarcoidosis ★★★★
Systemic lupus erythematosus ★★
Polyarteritis nodosa ★★
Tuberculosis ★★
Polymyalgia rheumatica ★
Systemic lupus erythematosus ★
Acquired immunodeficiency syndrome ★
The incubation period for acute brucellosis ranges from under two weeks to several months. During the acute illness, both liver and spleen may become enlarged. Laboratory tests include:
Granulopenia, with atypical lymphocytes;
Serological tests – standard agglutination, standard agglutination with added 2-mercapto-ethanol, antihuman globulin, complement fixation.

Case IV

1. CT scan of head ★★★★
Radioisotope brain scan ★★★★
Myelogram after CT scan ★★★★
Lumbar puncture after CT scan ★★★★

2. Sagittal vein thrombosis ★★★★
Spinal cord compression by extradural abscess ★★★★
Encephalitis ★★   Cerebral abscess ★
Sagittal sinus thrombosis may be a complication of severe dehydration, particularly in the infant, with diarrhoea. Obstruction of the sinus leads to cerebral swelling and raised intracranial pressure. If the thrombosis extends into the cortical veins, widespread haemorrhagic infarction of the brain may occur.

Case V

1. Cervical and dorsal spine X-rays ★★★★
Thoracolumbar myelogram ★★★★
Magnetic resonance imaging of spine ★★★★
Serum B12 and folate ★★
Technetium MDP bone scan ★★
Bone marrow aspirate ★★
VDRL TPHA ★

2. Spinal cord compression (D4) by tumour ★★★★
Spinal cord tumour ★★★★
Meningioma ★★
Subacute combined degeneration ★
Transverse myelitis ★   Tabes dorsalis ★
Anterior spinal artery occlusion ★

Answers

1. Left ventricular premature beats ★★★★
   ST segment ↓ in V₄, V₆, aVL ★★★★
   T wave inversion in I, V₆ ★★★★

2. 2:1 Second degree constant block ★★★★
   Mobitz type II block ★★★★
   This is a more severe A-V block than the periodic Mobitz type II block. In 2:1 second degree constant block, it is impossible to determine whether the block is in the A-V node (type I) or distal to the bundle of His (type II) without bundle of His recordings. This condition is an indication for pacing.

3. Nephrotic syndrome ★★★★
   Protein-losing state ★★★★
   Cirrhosis 0
   Myeloma 0
   The α_2 band is raised and the γ zone reduced. α_2 bands are typically raised in nephrotic syndrome, with reduction of other fractions. These findings would be characteristic for the nephrotic syndrome and other protein-losing states.

4. (a) Recurrent 'focal' glomerulonephritis ★★★★
       (syn.: Berger's nephritis, IgG-IgA nephritis)
       Henoch-Schoenlein purpura ★★
       Papillary necrosis ★
       Post-streptococcal glomerulonephritis 0
   (b) Renal biopsy ★★★★
       Serum IgA estimation ★★★★
       Immune complex estimation ★★★★
       Intravenous urogram ★★
       Urine culture ★★
   This may be the commonest cause of glomerular disease in Europe and Australia. The typical lesion, by light microscopy, consists of a focal glomerulonephritis. It is also segmental with lesions seen in some glomerular tufts but not others. Immune deposits are present diffusely in the mesangium of all glomeruli and contain IgA as the predominant immunoglobulin. The condition is three times more common in males, most cases presenting before the age of 35. Gross haematuria may occur, coincident with, or shortly after, a viral respiratory tract infection or influenza.

5. (a) Premature ovarian failure ★★★★
       Resistant ovary syndrome ★★
       Turner's syndrome 0
   (b) Pergonal stimulation test ★★★★
       Laparoscopic ovarian biopsy ★★★★
       Ovarian autoantibodies ★★★★
       Karyotype ★★★★
       Buccal smear ★
   The association of elevated basal gonadotrophins with an inappropriately low serum oestradiol is diagnostic of primary gonadal failure. Causes include autoimmune oophoritis, and chromosomal abnormalities such as the triple-x and isochromosome-x syndromes. If elevated gonadotrophins are found in the presence of normal oestrogen production, the patient may be suffering from the 'resistant ovary syndrome'. In this condition, ovarian histology shows oocytes and follicles (usually of abnormal appearance), and patients do not usually ovulate or increase their oestrogen output during gonadotrophin treatment. In this condition, spontaneous recovery (and pregnancy) may occur.

6. (a) Salicylate poisoning ★★★★
       Lactic acidosis ★★
   (b) Salicylate estimation ★★★★
       Plasma electrolytes ★★★★
   The ferric chloride test suggests the presence of a reducing sugar in the urine. With hypoglycaemia this is unlikely to be glucose. The metabolic acidosis of salicylate intoxication develops largely because of the interference of aspirin with carbohydrate, lipid, protein and amino acid metabolism. Serum lactic and pyruvic acids rise because of inhibition of Kreb's cycle enzymes. Fat metabolism is stimulated with production of ketone bodies.

7. (a) Acute cold haemagglutinin disease ★★★★
       Autoimmune haemolytic anaemia ★★
       Intravascular haemolysis ★★
       Haemolytic anaemia ★
   (b) Haemoglobinuria ★★★★
   The features suggest an acute intravascular haemolysis, in the aftermath of a viral infection. This may occur secondary to the production of 'cold' antibodies, which are active against the blood group antigens P, I, i (and other substances). The antibody is always IgM, with kappa light chains only. Complement is fixed and intravascular haemolysis occurs.

8. Myasthenia gravis ★★★★
   Opiate narcosis ★★★★   Asthma ★
   This was the vitalograph tracing of a patient with myasthenia gravis before and after intravenous edrophonium chloride (10mg). An alternative possibility is the effect of i.v. naloxone in a patient with opiate narcosis.

9. (a) Electrolyte estimation ★★★★
       Fibrin degradation products ★★★★
       Blood film to look for schistocytes ★★★★
       Plasma haemoglobin level ★★
       Methaemalbumin level ★★
       Urinary haemoglobin ★★
       Fibrinogen level ★★
       Urine microscopy for casts ★★
       Creatinine clearance ★
   (b) Haemolytic uraemic syndrome (HUS) ★★★★
       Microangiopathic haemolytic anaemia ★★★★
       Henoch-Schonlein purpura ★★
   HUS usually follows a febrile illness associated with diarrhoea which is often bloody. Intravascular haemolysis is followed by oliguria. Purpura, bleeding, drowsiness, anaemia and hypertension may occur. The peripheral blood film shows schistocytes and occasional spherocytes, thrombocytopenia, and usually leucocytosis. Treatment consists of supportive care, transfusion, hydration, control of hypertension and, if necessary, dialysis. If oliguria is prolonged, the chances of chronic renal damage occurring are greater.

10. (a) Left renal vein thrombosis ★★★★
        Renal artery embolus ★★★★
    (b) Renal renogram ★★★★
        Intravenous urography ★★★★
        Radioisotope renogram ★★★★
        Ultrasound of kidneys ★★
    Renal vein thrombosis is a complication of the hypercoagulable state present in the nephrotic syndrome. Thromboses, both arterial and venous, are common in this condition. Hypercoagulability has multiple aetiologies: fibrinogen and factor VIII are increased, while anti-thrombin III is lost in the urine, and plasminogen activator release and tissue fibrinolysis are reduced. The haematocrit may also be raised. For unknown reasons, patients with amyloidosis, membranous nephropathy and mesangiocapillary glomerulonephritis are particularly susceptible to this complication of the nephrotic syndrome.

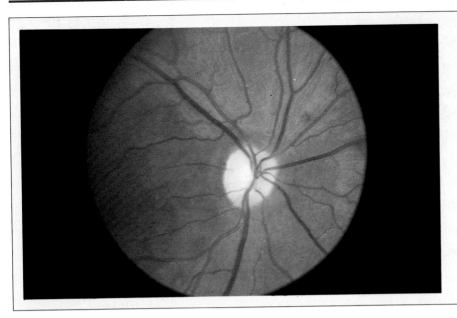

1. (a) What is the diagnosis?
   (b) List four possible causes.

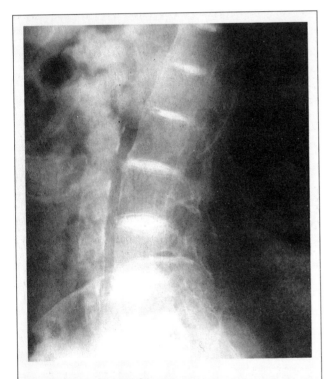

2. What is the diagnosis?

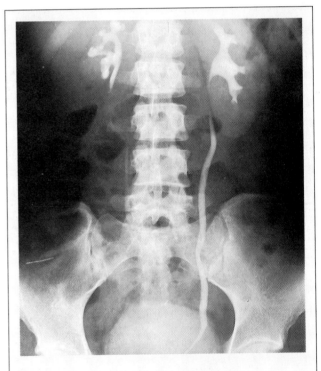

3. (a) List three abnormalities on this excretory urogram.
   (b) What is the likely underlying diagnosis?

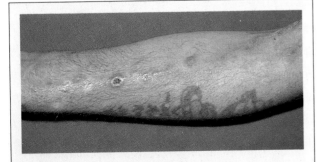

4. (a) What is the likely cause of this appearance?
   (b) Suggest a further possible diagnosis.

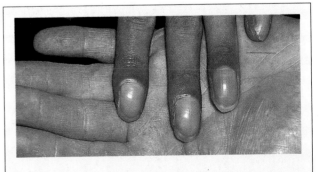

5. Suggest two possible causes for this appearance.

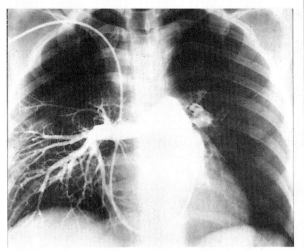

6. (a) What is the investigation?
(b) What is the diagnosis?

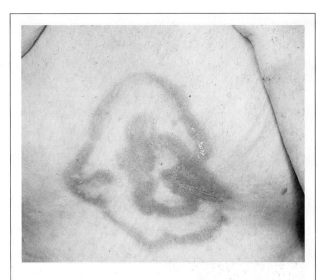

7. This lesion was found on the trunk of a 65-year-old woman with known carcinoma of the breast.
What is the diagnosis?

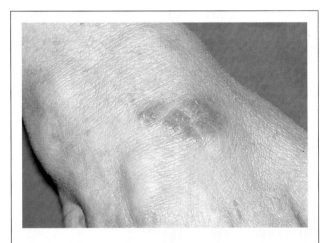

8. This lesion appeared insidiously in a 65-year-old woman. It had started as a painless deep nodule and slowly formed a plaque as it coalesced with neighbouring lesions within a few weeks.
Suggest two possible diagnoses.

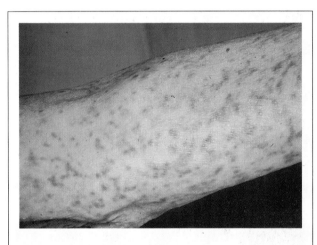

9. This patient's eruption itched after a hot bath or when the skin was scratched.
What is the diagnosis?

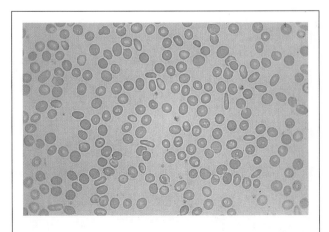

10. (a) List four abnormalities present on this blood film.
(b) What is the likely diagnosis?

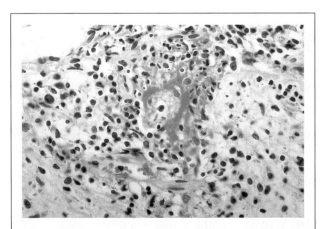

11. This is the skin biopsy from a man presenting with fever, weight loss and multiple gangrenous lesions on his arms.
What is the diagnosis?

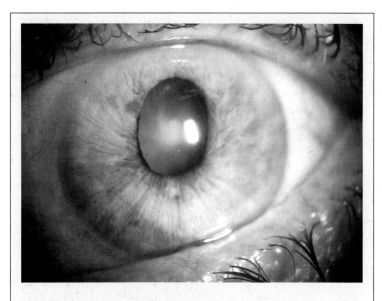

12. (a) What two abnormalities are present?
(b) What is the likely diagnosis?

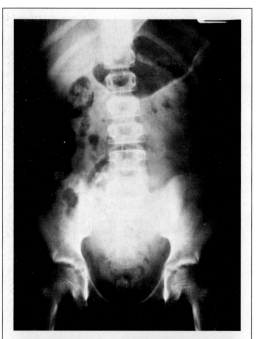

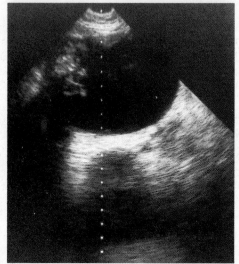

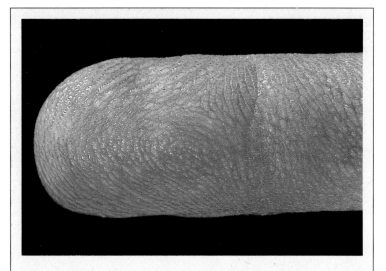

13. With what skin condition is this fingerprint abnormality associated?

14. This is the abdominal radiograph and pelvic ultrasound of a 20-year-old female.
(a) What abnormality is shown?
(b) What is the diagnosis?

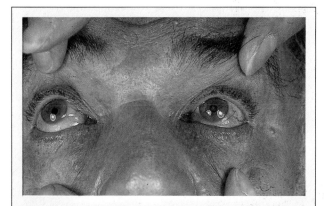

15. What is the diagnosis?

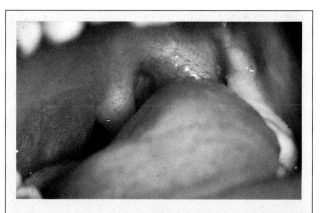

16. This abnormality appeared four days after the onset of a severe sore throat.
What is the most likely diagnosis?

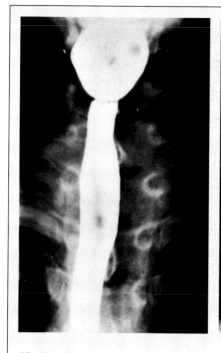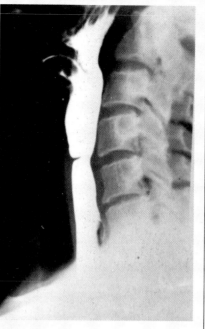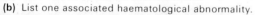

17. This 50-year-old woman complained of intermittent dysphagia for solid foods.
    (a) What does her barium swallow show?
    (b) List one associated haematological abnormality.

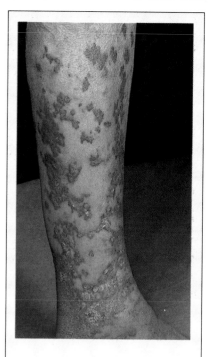

18. What is the cause of these chronic lesions?

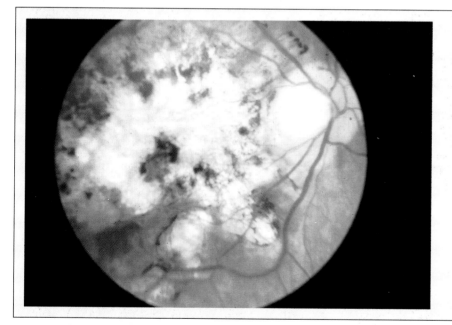

19. List four possible causes for this fundal appearance.

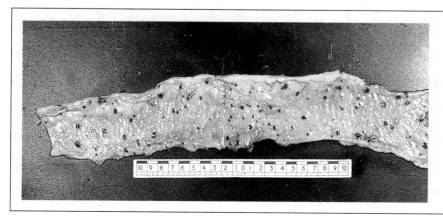

20. What is the likely cause of the appearance of this post-mortem small bowel specimen?

Case Histories

CASE I

A 16-year old Turkish girl presented with a short history of becoming withdrawn. For some days before, she had apparently been excitable and exhibiting outbursts of violent behaviour, which was totally out of character. She had been well in the past, except for an episode nine months before, when she had developed aches and pains in her joints and some swelling of the knee and wrist joints. During that time she had vomited and experienced non-specific pains in the chest which were sometimes pleuritic in nature. These symptoms were treated with aspirin and they remitted after ten days or so. Her GP had at that time noticed some thinning of her scalp hair and a trace of proteinuria on urine testing, but after retesting a week later, her urine had become clear.

On examination, the patient was conscious but withdrawn. She would not utter any words or obey commands. Periodically, her eyes moved conjugately. She seemed unable to fix any target for more than a brief period of time. There were no spontaneous movements, although, if lifted out of bed, she would stand. She would indefinitely maintain any posture into which her limbs were placed. Pulse 65/min regular, blood pressure 120/70mmHg. Cardiac auscultation revealed an ejection systolic murmur audible at the apex, but no other abnormalities. Her lungs were clear and abdominal examination was normal with no tenderness or masses present. She was apyrexial. The central nervous system examination revealed soft exudates present in both fundi, but the remainder of the cranial nerves were normal except for her mutism. Reflexes appeared to be brisk, and the right plantar was equivocal with a left flexor response. Residual scalp alopecia was noted.

Investigations

HAEMATOLOGY
Hb: 9.1g/dl (9.1g/100ml); WBC: 8.2×10⁹/l (8,200/mm3); Platelets: 250 × 10⁹/l (250,000/mm3); Reticulocytes: 3.8%; ESR: 132mm/h.

BIOCHEMISTRY
Urea: 3.6mmol/l (22mg/100ml); Sodium: 140mmol/l (140mEq/l); Potassium: 4.7mmol/l (4.7mEq/l); Bicarbonate: 27mmol/l (27mEq/l); Chloride: 98mmol/l (98mEq/l); Bilirubin: 14μmol/l (0.82mg/100ml); Alkaline phosphatase: 140 iu/l (18 KAU/100ml); Total protein: 72g/l (7.2g/100ml); Albumin: 34g/l (3.4g/100ml); Calcium: 2.5mmol/l (9.9mg/100ml); Serum glutamic oxaloacetic transaminase (SGOT): 33iu/l; Uric acid: 0.33mmol/l (5.5mg/100ml); Complement C3 level: 31iu/ml (normal range: 71–154iu/ml).

RADIOLOGY
CXR: normal cardiac contour, no parenchymal shadowing; ECG: within normal limits; CT scan of head: widening of the cortical sulci is noted, with a small ill-defined, non-enhancing low attenuation lesions in the parietal and temporal regions of both hemispheres.

1. List three investigations which would be diagnostically useful.

2. What is the most likely diagnosis?

CASE II

A 55-year-old housewife was admitted as an emergency because of a sudden onset of left hypochondrial pain. The pain had started suddenly whilst she was watching television, and had become progressively worse, exacerbated by deep inspiration and coughing. There was no haemoptysis. She had been well in the past, and apart from a course of antidepressants two years before, following the death of her husband, she took no regular medication. For six months, she had noticed increasing breathlessness particularly on negotiating the two flights of stairs to her flat. She had, however, put these symptoms down to her age and to the fact that she had put on some weight.

On examination, she looked distressed and her skin was clammy. Her pulse was irregular 120/min and her blood pressure was 110/70mmHg. There was no lymphadenopathy, and auscultation of the lung fields was clear. However, she appeared to be splinting her respiration and was not expanding the left lower chest during deep inspiration. There was tenderness overlying the ninth, tenth and eleventh ribs in the axilla. Cardiac auscultation revealed a loud first sound and a low-pitched diastolic murmur best heard at the apex. There was no organomegaly in the abdomen, although the left hypochondrium was tender. The rest of the clinical examination was unremarkable.

Investigations

Hb: 11.6g/dl (11.6g/100ml); MCV: 83fl (83μm3); WBC: 6.9×10⁹/l (6,900//mm3); Normal differential count; ESR: 27mm/h; Urea and electrolytes: normal; Liver function tests: normal; PA CXR: double right heart border, splaying of the carina and elevation of the left main bronchus; ECG: coarse atrial fibrillation waves seen; Urinanalysis: trace proteinuria.

1. List two investigations which would be useful at this stage.

2. What is the most likely underlying diagnosis?

CASE III

A 52-year-old man was brought to Casualty as an emergency because of onset of headache and drowsiness. His wife said that he had been well until two hours before admission, when he developed a sudden headache affecting mainly the back of the head. This had been exceedingly severe and had caused him to vomit. Shortly after the onset of the headache he had lost consciousness for a short period of time, but upon regaining consciousness he complained of double vision in virtually all directions of gaze. His wife remarked that his speech appeared very slurred, as if he was drunk, and that his arms, particularly his left side, were very clumsy. He was unable to reach out for a cup of tea, and seemed to have great difficulty with bringing the cup to his lips. Shortly afterwards the patient once again became drowsy, and his GP referred him straight to hospital. In his medical history, apart from mild hypertension treated with a beta-blocker, he had been well. As a child he had had his tonsils and adenoids removed. He had smoked 20 cigarettes each day for the last 13 years. His wife also said that he drank three to four pints of beer in the evenings and had occasionally come home drunk.

On examination, the patient was pyrexial at 37.5°C. Miosis was present. He was clearly drowsy, but when questioned he seemed moderately well orientated in time and place. There was nystagmus in virtually all directions of gaze and his speech was dysarthric. Finger to nose testing was clumsy, particularly on the left. Reflexes were brisk in all four limbs, and the jaw jerk was brisk.

1. Give two steps which should be taken in his immediate management.

2. What is the most likely diagnosis?

CASE IV

A 38-year-old woman presented to her GP with a four month history of loss of scalp hair, headaches and irritability. Although her general health had been good in the past, it was noted that she had had hypochondriacal tendencies from a young age. A benzodiazapine was prescribed, but her symptoms failed to subside, and she later presented with gradual onset of anorexia associated with occasional vomiting and a 4kg weight loss. She also complained that her skin was becoming dry and scaly. On referral, she admitted to being of an anxious disposition, and over the last three years she had taken to a strict vegetarian diet. She ascribed most illnesses to dietary causes, and strongly believed that a high intake of vegetables conferred beneficial powers. She took no medication other than pills from a health stall. In her family history it was noted that a younger brother suffered from epilepsy, and that her father had committed suicide because of depression.

On examination, she appeared pale with evidence of diffuse capital alopecia. Temperature was 37°C. There was no temporal recession. Her skin appeared dry and there was no lymphadeno-pathy. Pulse 80/min regular, blood pressure 110/75mmHg. Examination of the heart and lungs was normal. In the abdomen, a three finger smooth, non-tender enlargement of the liver was noted. She was dull to percussion in the left hypochondrium, and the tip of the spleen could just be felt. The rest of the abdominal examination was unremarkable. Fundal examination revealed fullness of the optic discs, with loss of venous pulsation. The retinal veins were dilated. Reflexes were symmetrical but brisk, and plantars were bilaterally flexor.

Investigations

HAEMATOLOGY
Hb: 11.6g/dl (11.6g/100ml); MCV: 82fl (82μm^3); WBC: 5.9×10^9/l (5,900/mm^3); Normal differential count; ESR: 30mm/h.

BIOCHEMISTRY & RADIOLOGY
Urea: 5.2mmol/l (32mg/100ml); Sodium: 138mmol/l (138mEq/l); Potassium: 4.7mmol/l (4.7mEq/l); Bicarbonate: 25mmol/l (25mEq/l); Chloride: 101mmol/l (101mEq/l); Bilirubin: 21μmol/l (1.2mg/100ml); Alkaline phosphatase: 135iu/l (17.5KAU/100ml); Total protein: 70g/l (7.0g/100ml); Albumin: 37g/l (3.7g/100ml); Calcium: 2.42mmol/l (9.5mg/100ml); Phosphate: 0.94mmol/l (3.4mg/100ml); SGOT: 57iu/l; Serum hydroxybutyrate dehydrogenase (HBD): 111iu/l; Urinanalysis: normal; CXR: normal; ECG: Sinus rhythm normal QRS complexes and no repolarisation abnormalities.

1. What is the most likely diagnosis?

2. What further investigations would be useful?

CASE V

A 56-year-old woman was investigated because of frequent blood-stained faeces and severe iron deficiency anaemia. She had been in good health until five weeks before, when she passed fresh blood per rectum. Bleeding recurred four times over the next two weeks. She attributed all her symptoms to haemorrhoids. Two weeks later the bleeding recurred, but it was not associated with change of bowel habit, and there was no mucus in the stool. In the past, she had suffered from osteoarthritis for ten years and was under treatment for hypothyroidism. During the last two years, she had complained of diffuse abdominal pains unrelated to meals, which had been ascribed to irritable bowel. There was no history of aspirin ingestion or alcohol abuse, and she had not lost weight or appetite.

On examination, her temperature was 36.3°C, pulse 80/min regular, blood pressure 160/80mmHg. The patient looked well, although a little pale. Examination of the head and neck was normal, but cardiac auscultation revealed a harsh systolic ejection murmur at the cardiac apex through to the base, with radiation to both carotid arteries. A grade II decrescendo diastolic murmur was audible at the left sternal edge. The liver and spleen were not palpable, and no mass was found in the abdomen. Neurological examination was unremarkable.

Investigations

HAEMATOLOGY
Hb: 7.4g/dl (7.4g/100ml); MCV: 64fl (64μm^3); MCH: 19pg (19$\mu\mu$g); WBC: 9.1×10^9/l (9,100/mm^3); Platelets: 347×10^9/l (347,000/mm^3); Reticulocytes: 3.4%; ESR: 10mm/h.

BIOCHEMISTRY & RADIOLOGY
Electrolytes: normal; Urea: 8.9mmol/l (54mg/100ml); Glucose: 6.9mmol/l (124mg/100ml); Liver function tests: normal; Urinanalysis: normal; CXR: mild enlargement of the cardiac silhouette with prominent left ventricle, lung fields clear; Abdominal X-ray: normal; ECG: some non-specific ST segment and T wave abnormalities seen; Barium enema examination: normal; Barium swallow: normal.

1. List three investigations which would be diagnostically useful.

2. Give two possible diagnoses.

Data Interpretations

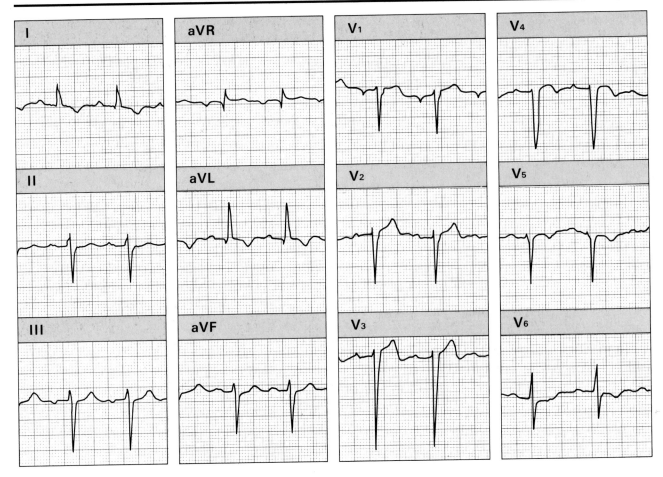

1. List three abnormalities on this ECG.

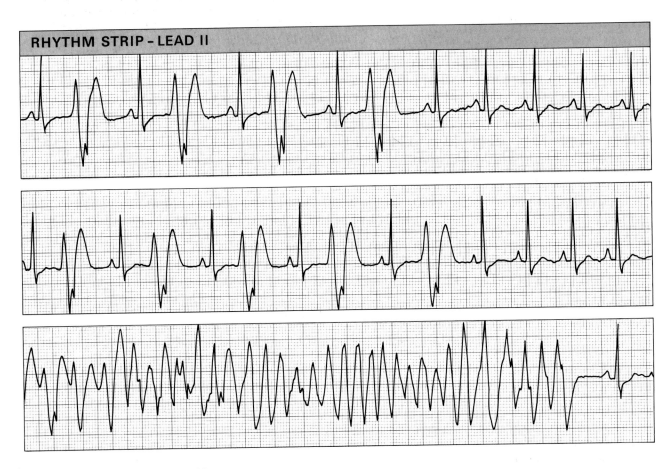

7.8 2. List three abnormalities on this ECG.

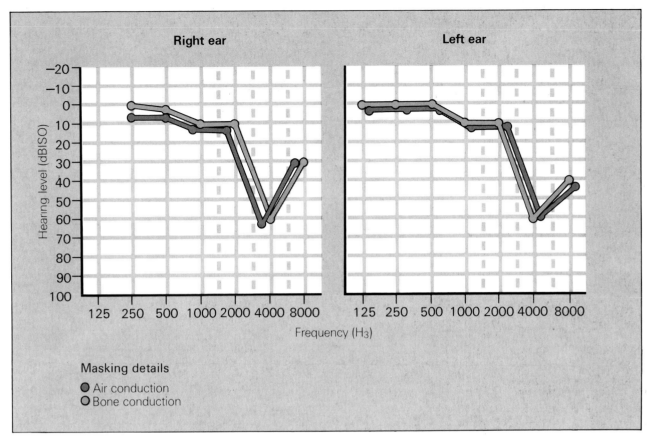

Right ear

Left ear

Hearing level (dBISO)

Frequency (H₃)

Masking details
- ● Air conduction
- ○ Bone conduction

3. What is the most likely cause of this audiometric appearance?

4. A 28-year-old woman is investigated because of breathlessness.
Lung function: VC: 2.33l (predicted 2.4–3.6); FEV₁: 1.35l; FIV₁: 1.65l; RV: 2.89l (predicted 1.55–2.32); FRC: 3.56l (predicted 2.17–3.25); TLC: 5.89l (predicted 3.96–5.66); TLCO: 4.7mmol/min/kPa (predicted 5.8–8.7); KCO: 0.98mmol/min/kPa/l.
(a) What is the most likely diagnosis?
(b) Suggest two possible causes.

5. A 55-year-old man presents with central abdominal pain and vomiting. He has lost over 10kg in body weight over three months. A succussion splash is present.
Sodium: 132mmol/l (132mEq/l); Potassium: 3.1mmol/l (3.1mEq/l); Chloride: 84mmol/l (84mEq/l); Urea: 16.4mmol/l (99mg/100ml).
What is the most likely diagnosis based on the above findings?

6. A 38-year-old woman is admitted severely breathless.
Arterial gases on room air: pH: 7.39; PaO₂: 8.02kPa (60mmHg); PaCO₂: 2.9kPa (22mmHg); Bicarbonate: 13mmol/l (13mEq/l); BEB: −12; SatO₂: 89%.
List three possible causes.

7. A 35-year-old woman undergoes a pentagastrin test. After an overnight fast, a one hour basal secretion of acid is 1.2mmol of hydrogen ion. After 6μg/kg pentagastrin intramuscularly, 4 ×15min gastric aspirates were examined.

Sample	pH
1	3.9
2	3.7
3	3.6
4	3.8

(a) What is the diagnosis?
(b) Suggest a possible cause.

8. A 45-year-old diabetic patient, usually well controlled on oral hypoglycaemics, is admitted severely dehydrated.
Sodium: 148mmol/l (148mEq/l); Potassium: 3.2mmol/l (3.2mEq/l); Bicarbonate: 4mmol/l (4mEq/l); Chloride: 118mmol/l (118mEq/l); PaCO₂: 1.8kPa (13.5mmHg); pH: 7.08; Glucose: 7.8mmol/l (140mg/100ml); Urea: 14.8mmol/l.
(a) What abnormality is demonstrated?
(b) Suggest a possible cause for this patient's condition.

9. A 45-year-old woman is investigated for lethargy and weakness. A long synacthen test (1mg depot synacthen s/c) is carried out.

Time (h)	Cortisol (nmol/l)
0	150
0.30	155
1	170
4	260
8	370
24	745

(a) What is the most likely diagnosis?
(b) Suggest two further diagnostically useful investigations.

10. A 64-year-old woman gives a long history of anorexia and weakness.
Calcium: 3.01mmol/l (11.9mg/100ml); Phosphate: 0.8mmol/l (2.6mg/100ml); Albumin: 43g/l (4.3g/100ml); Alkaline phosphatase: 135iu/l; Sodium: 136mmol/l (136mEq/l); Potassium: 3.3mmol/l (3.3mEq/l); Chloride: 113mmol/l (113mEq/l); Bicarbonate: 21mmol/l (21mEq/l); Urea: 6.7mmol/l (35mg/100ml); ESR: 8mm/h.
(a) List four investigations which would assist in the diagnosis.
(b) What is the probable diagnosis?

Answers

1. **(a)** Optic atrophy in a negroid fundus ★★★★
       Optic atrophy ★★
   (b) Retrobulbar neuritis ★★★★
       Optic nerve compression ★★★★
       Trauma or ischaemia ★★★★
       Toxins (methanol, tobacco) ★★★★
       B1 or B12 deficiency ★★★★
       Neurosyphilis ★★★★
       Hereditary optic atrophy (Leber's) ★★★★
       Friedreich's ataxia ★★★★

2. Alkaptonuria ★★★★
   Osteoporosis ★★★
   Calcification of the intervertebral discs and osteopenia is present, as evidenced by the prominent vertical trabeculae seen particularly in the low lumbar vertebrae. Calcification of the aorta is also present. These are the characteristic signs of alkaptonuria (see p.11.2).

3. **(a)** Abnormalities reside in the right kidney:
       Small right kidney ★★★★
       Thinning of the renal cortex ★★★★
       Dilated calyces ★★★★
       Clubbing of calyces ★★★★
   (b) Chronic pyelonephritis ★★★★
   This type of chronic non-obstructive pyelonephritic kidney is likely to result from previous infection in childhood. Post-infectious renal sclerosis and atrophy are most likely to occur in the growing kidney; such childhood infection is usually responsible for the discovery of a unilateral contracted kidney.

4. **(a)** Infected injection sites in a drug addict ★★★★
   (b) Sporotrichosis ★★★★
       Dermatitis artefacta ★
       Lichen striatus ★
       Linear psoriasis ★
       Cutaneous leishmaniasis 0
   Sporotrichosis is a chronic fungal infection usually localised to cutaneous lymphatic tissues, and caused by the dimorphic fungus *Sporothrix schenkii*. It frequently affects labourers, farmers and florists, and is considered a true occupational disease. In the lymphatic form of the disease, the earliest lesion is a pustule, papule or nodule which enlarges, becomes red or violaceous and is followed by a chain of subcutaneous nodules along regional lymphatics. These may ulcerate and drain a thin grey to yellow pus. The cutaneous lymphatic form responds to the oral administration of iodides.

5. Cyanotic heart disease ★★★★
   Fibrosing alveolitis ★★★★
   Cystic fibrosis ★★★★
   Bronchiectasis ★★★★
   There is clubbing with cyanosis.

6. **(a)** Pulmonary arteriogram ★★★★
       Cardiocatheter 0
   (b) Multiple pulmonary emboli ★★★★
   There is complete absence of vascular markings in the left lung, and in the upper lobe of the right lung consistent with massive pulmonary emboli.

7. Annular erythema ★★★★
   Erythema gyratum repens ★★★★
   Erythema annulare centrifugum ★★★★
   Annular psoriasis ★
   Tinea incognito ★
   Erythema gyratum repens consists of irregular wavy bands with peculiar gyrate or serpiginous outline, with marginal desquamation of the trunk, neck and extremities. It is associated with carcinoma of the breast, tongue or lung.

8. Lupus vulgaris ★★★★
   Cutaneous sarcoidosis ★★★★
   Secondary deposits in the skin ★★
   Cutaneous leishmaniasis ★★
   Lymphocytoma cutis ★
   Cutaneous tuberculosis is grouped into two categories. The first, in which organisms are present, includes lupus vulgaris, tuberculosis verrucosa cutis, scrofuloderma (skin changes surrounding a draining tuberculous sinus or overlying a tuberculous node), and tuberculosis orificialis. The second group comprises the tuberculides and includes Bazin's erythema induratum, an allergic condition.

9. Urticaria pigmentosa ★★★★
   Mastocytosis ★★★★
   The lesions of urticaria pigmentosa when stroked will produce a wheal (Darier's sign). Urticaria pigmentosa occurs primarily in children, when it runs a benign course. When it occurs in adults, non-cutaneous organ involvement must be suspected. When selecting a site for biopsy, this should not be stroked, in case the granules are discharged from the cells. Histologically, the nest of mast cells is diagnostic.

10. **(a)** Anisocytosis ★★★★
        Poikilocytosis ★★★★
        Microcytosis ★★★★
        Hypochromia ★★★★
        Pencil cells ★★★★
        Target cells ★★★★
    (b) Severe iron deficiency anaemia ★★★★
    The presence of pencil cells, the target cells and the hypochromia are characteristic of severe iron deficiency anaemia.

11. Polyarteritis nodosa ★★★★
    Necrotising vasculitis ★★★★
    Thrombophlebitis 0
    The section shows features of a necrotising arteriolitis, with evidence of oedema, fibrinous exudation, fibrinoid necrosis and infiltration of polymorphonuclear neutrophils in the wall of the vessel.

12. **(a)** Corneal clouding secondary to oedema ★★★★
        Oval shape-mid dilated pupil ★★★★
        Arcus senilis ★★★★
        Eye post-mydriatic ★
    (b) Acute closed angle glaucoma ★★★★
    Acute closed angle glaucoma is associated with severe pain and rapid onset of visual impairment. The increased intraocular pressure (normally 10–21mmHg) leads to paralysis of the papillary sphincter muscle, resulting in a fixed, mid dilated pupil. Ciliary injection is usually present. The disease is caused by mechanical blockage of the outflow channels in the angle, by the iris coming into contact with the trabecular meshwork. Vision is blurred or foggy, and coloured halos are seen around lights, as the cornea assumes a steamy appearance (oedema).

13. Acanthosis nigricans ★★★★
    The fingerprint is verrucous.

14. **(a)** There is a pelvic mass which is largely cystic in nature with echogenic areas within it ★★★★
        Cystic mass ★★
    (b) Cystic teratoma (dermoid cyst) ★★★★
        Ovarian cyst ★★
    These lesions commonly contain teeth, making diagnosis easy. On ultrasound, acoustic shadowing is frequently demonstrated, more commonly associated with hair and sebum than with calcification or osseous elements.

15. Argyrosis ★★★★

The pigmented appearances over the caruncula are due to silver nitrate deposition; the patient had been using silver nitrate eye drops. This appearance is quite different from those in ochronosis, or osteogenesis imperfecta, where lesions are confined to the sclera.

16. Quinsy ★★★★

Peritonsillar abscess ★★★★
Lymphoma of tonsil 0
This results from a streptococcal pharyngitis. Suppuration extends through the capsule of the palatine tonsil into the adjacent loose connective tissue. The involved tonsil and anterior pillar are greatly swollen, and the ipsilateral cervical nodes are large and tender. The pus does not regularly contain streptococci, but may permit commensal organisms such as anaerobic Gram-negative bacilli of the oropharynx and anaerobic non-haemolytic streptococci to gain a foothold in the affected tissues.

17. Cricopharyngeal web ★★★★

Iron deficiency anaemia ★★★★
These appearances are associated with iron deficiency anaemia – the Plummer-Vinson or Paterson-Kelly syndrome. Previously there was thought to be an increased risk of squamous cell carcinoma, although this is currently disputed.

18. Kaposi's sarcoma ★★★★

These are the appearances of classical Kaposi's sarcoma. The lesions may be single or multiple patches, plaques, or tumours occurring on the lower legs and associated usually with chronic oedema. The lesions are usually a violaceous or purple colour, and are associated with burst post-inflammatory pigmentation.

19. Congenital:

Toxoplasmosis ★★★★
Sarcoidosis ★★★★
Syphilis ★★★★
Toxocara ★★★★
Behçet's disease ★★★★
Idiopathic ★★
Ocular histoplasmosis ★
Systemic lupus erythematosus ★
Diabetes mellitus – post-photocoagulation ★
In congenital toxoplasmosis there are bilateral and frequently multiple choroidoretinal lesions, the macula being particularly involved. The whole thickness of the retina and choroid is destroyed in a necrotising inflammation so that a punched-out, heavily pigmented scar remains. In infants, the infection is frequently associated with an encephalitis.

20. Malignant melanoma ★★★★

Melanosis coli 0
This is a classical site of visceral metastatic spread of malignant melanoma.

ANSWERS TO CASE HISTORIES

Case I

1. Antinuclear factor ★★★★
   Double-stranded DNA antibodies ★★★★
   EEG ★★★★
   CRP ('C' reactive protein) ★★★★
   Serological testing for syphilis ★★
   CSF examination ★★
   Search for LE cells ★★
   CH50 estimation ★
   C4 estimation ★
   Anti-Sm (present in 25% of cases) ★
   Anti-Ro ★

2. Cerebral lupus erythematosus ★★★★
   Viral encephalitis ★★
   Behcet's disease ★★
   Tuberculous meningitis ★
   Multifocal leucoencephalopathy 0
   Organic brain damage in systemic lupus erythematosus occurs in up to 15% of patients. The manifestations are varied, and include behavioural disturbance, hyperirritability, confusion, hallucinations, obsessional and paranoid reactions and frank organic psychosis. The latter may be difficult to differentiate from a steroid-induced psychosis. Other manifestations include convulsions (16%), peripheral neuropathy, hemiparesis, motor aphasia, ptosis, diplopia and nystagmus. CSF findings would be those of an aseptic meningitis.

Case II

1. Echocardiogram ★★★★
   Ventilation perfusion scan of the lungs ★★★★
   Technetium scan of liver and spleen ★★★★
   Blood gases ★★★★
   Blood cultures ★★★★
   Left lateral chest X-ray ★★
   Phonocardiogram ★

2. Splenic infarct from arterial embolus secondary to mitral stenosis ★★★★
   Pulmonary infarct ★★★★
   Long term anticoagulation is indicated in this case, as the risk of re-embolisation is greatly increased in the presence of atrial fibrillation, even when the mitral stenosis is mild.

Case III

1. CT scan of head ★★★★
   Urgent surgical exploration of posterior fossa to relieve cerebellar haematoma ★★★★
   Arteriographic study (vertebral arteriograms) ★★
   EEG 0
   Lumbar puncture 0

2. Cerebellar bleed with haematoma ★★★★
   Ruptured aneurysm with sub-arachnoid haemorrhage ★★★★
   Cerebral haemorrhage (right hemisphere) with secondary brainstem compression ★★★★
   Pontine haemorrhage ★★
   Wernicke's encephalopathy 0
   Intracerebellar haemorrhage is characterised by sudden severe occipital headache, diplopia, nystagmus and ataxia. On examination, the patient usually has miotic pupils, conjugate gaze palsies and irregular respiration. In some cases, the clinical features may have been present for several hours before any loss of consciousness, whereas in others loss of consciousness may be immediate. In contrast, brainstem haemorrhage usually causes immediate loss of consciousness, irregular respiration, pin point pupils and quadriplegia followed by rapid decline to death.

Case IV

1. Vitamin A intoxication ★★★★
   Malabsorption syndrome ★
   Hypothyroidism ★

2. Serum Vitamin A level ★★★★
   Fat absorption tests ★★
   Thyroid function tests ★★
   Prothrombin time ★★
   Fluorescein angiogram ★
   CT scan of head ★
   Bone marrow examination ★
   Liver biopsy ★
   Protein electrophoresis ★
   Acute hypervitaminosis A may cause drowsiness, irritability and severe vomiting within a few hours of ingestion. In children, chronic hypervitaminosis A has been reported to cause

hepatosplenomegaly, hypoplastic anaemia, leucopenia, precocious skeletal development, finger clubbing and coarse sparse hairs. In adults, there is an association with benign intracranial hypertension.

Case V

1. Small bowel enema ★★★★
   Colonoscopy ★★★★
   Rectal biopsy ★★
   Arteriogram during a bleed ★★
   Technetium scan to detect source of bleed ★★
   Meckel's scan ★★
   Bleeding time ★★
   Prothrombin time ★★
   Partial thromboplastin time ★★

2. Angiodysplasia ★★★★
   Aortic valve disease ★★★★
   Bleeding diathesis ★★
   Ischaemic colitis ★★
   Ulcerative colitis ★
   Crohn's disease ★
   Bleeding diverticulum ★
   Angiodysplastic lesions consist of ectatic areas of the mucosal microvasculature, especially the capillaries and venules, associated with dilatation of submucosal verns. There is an association with aortic stenosis. The lesions are best diagnosed by colonoscopy. They are not associated with cutaneous vascular lesions or lesions in other viscera. This is in contrast with the telangiectatic lesions of Rendu-Osler-Weber disease and Turner's syndrome, which also occur in the G.I. tract and cause gastrointestinal bleeding.

ANSWERS TO DATA INTERPRETATIONS

1. First degree heart block ★★★★
   Left anterior hemiblock (left axis deviation) ★★★★
   Poor R wave progression V_1–V_4 ★★★★★
   Ischaemic changes in lateral leads ★★
   Left atrial hypertrophy ★★

2. Bigeminus rhythm with R on T ★★★★
   Ventrical tachycardia ★★★★
   Ventricular fibrillation ★★★★
   There is a run of bigeminus rhythm followed by three sinus rhythm beats, followed by a bust of ventricular tachycardia which disintegrates into VF.

3. Noise-induced hearing loss ★★★★
   There is high frequency sensory-neural deafness, with a 4 kilohertz dip. This may be due to machine or gunfire damage.

4. (a) Obstruction of airways with underlying emphysema ★★★★
       Asthma ★
   (b) α_1-antitrypsin deficiency (homozygous) ★★★★
       Cigarette smoking ★★★★
       Cadmium poisoning (chronic inhalation of industrial fumes) ★★★★
       Bullous disease of the lung ★★
       McLeod's syndrome ★
       The FEV_1/FVC ratio is 58%. The total lung capacity is increased, as is the residual volume and functional residual capacity, and the RV/TLC is markedly increased. These are the features of obstructive airways disease. The markedly reduced TLCO is characteristic of emphysema.

5. Pyloric stenosis ★★★★
   Gastric carcinoma with pyloric obstruction ★★★★

Recurrent vomiting of gastric juice ★★★★
In pyloric stenosis, an excess of unbuffered H^+ is lost, together with chloride, leading to hypochloraemia. Chloride depletion may *per se* aggravate the metabolic alkalosis by preventing sodium reabsorption. Further, the low GFR caused by the accompanying water depletion reduces urinary bicarbonate loss which would otherwise tend to correct the alkalosis. Hypokalaemia occurs via urinary potassium loss.

6. Pulmonary embolus ★★★★
   Pulmonary oedema ★★★★
   Pneumonic consolidation ★★★★
   Moderately severe asthma ★★
   This pattern of arterial blood gases is compatible with a ventilation-perfusion defect (alveolar-capillary block), or an intrapulmonary right to left shunt. There is hypoxaemia and hypocapnia.

7. (a) Achlorydria ★★★★
   (b) Gastric atrophy ★★★★
       Campylobacter pyloridis gastritis ★★★★
       Chronic gastritis ★★
   Basal gastric acid secretion is 2.6±0.2mmol (mean ± 1SD) for males, and 1.6±0.2mmol for females. After maximal histamine or pentagastrin stimulation, there should be a ten-fold increase in output. Normal basal gastric pH is 0.9–1.5 in adults.

8. (a) Mixed anion gap/normal anion gap acidosis ★★★★
       Hyperchloraemic acidosis ★★
       Lactic acidosis ★★
   (b) Phenformin-induced lactic acidosis ★★★★
   The anion gap (AG) is 29.8mmol/l (normally 15mmol/l), giving a $\triangle$ AG of 14.8mmol/l. However, the $\triangle$ HCO_3^- (normally bicarbonate is $\simeq$ 25mmol/l) is 21mmol/l, therefore this is not a pure anion gap acidosis (where the ratio $\triangle AG/\triangle HCO_3^-$ would be $\simeq$ 1), but a mixed anion gap/normal anion gap acidosis. Hyperchloraemia is responsible for the mixed anion gap acidosis component.

9. (a) Secondary adrenocortical failure ★★★★
       Hypopituitarism ★★★★
       Addison's disease 0
   (b) X-ray of pituitary fossa ★★★★
       T4 estimation ★★★★
       Assessment of basal and dynamic pituitary function ★★★★
       CT scan of pituitary hypothalamic region ★★★★
       Skull X-ray ★★
       Plasma/urine osmolality ★★
   The gradual increase in cortisol following 1mg of depot synacthen is typical of secondary adrenal insufficiency, the peak control occurring at 24 hours. A normal cortisol response to depot synacthen would yield a peak at 2–4 hours.

10. (a) Plasma PTH estimation ★★★★
        Hydrocortisone suppression test ★★★★
        Macro-X-ray of hand (subperiosteal erosions) ★★★★
        Urinary calcium estimation ★★★★
        CT scan of neck ★★
        Ultrasound of neck ★★
        Barium swallow to look for indentation of enlarged parathyroid on column of barium ★★
        Thallium/technetium substraction scan of parathyroids ★
    (b) Primary hyperparathyroidism ★★★★
        Myeloma 0
    The presence of hypophosphataemia, normal urea and ESR make hyperparathyroidism the most likely diagnosis. A urinary calcium estimation (with simultaneous creatinine clearance) will help to exclude hypercalcaemic hypocalciuria, a familial condition requiring no specific treatment.

Paper 8

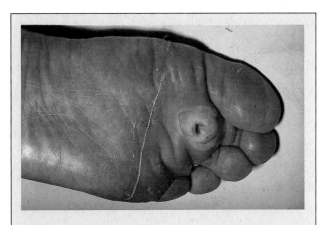

1. This lesion has been present for two months.
   What is the likely diagnosis?

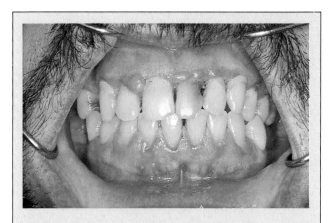

2. This man was under investigation for a chronic
   anaemia.
   Suggest an underlying diagnosis.

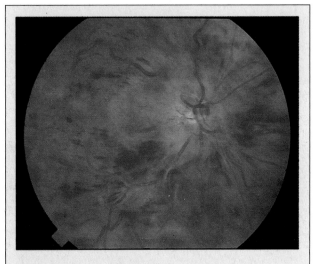

3. (a) What is the diagnosis?
   (b) List two predisposing causes.

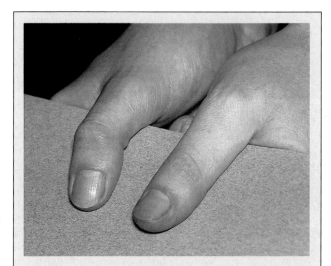

4. This patient was asked to grip the sheet of paper
   between the thumb and forefinger.
   What abnormality is shown?

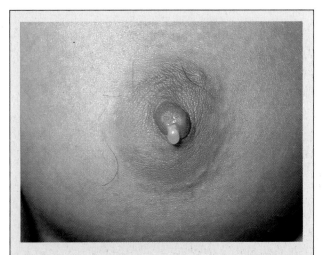

5. List three possible causes for this physical sign found
   in a non-post partum woman.

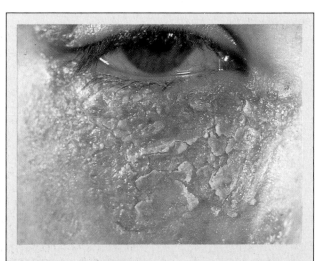

6. What is the diagnosis?

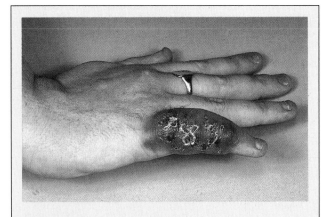

7. This chronic lesion was present in a 35-year-old woman with a long-standing eye disorder.
   (a) What is the most likely diagnosis?
   (b) List three ocular manifestations of this disorder.

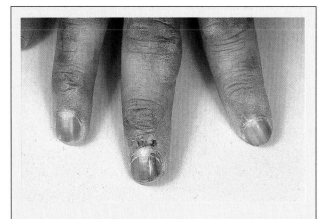

8. These are the fingers of a 26-year-old man, from Burma (now Myanmar). There are several apparently painless traumatic areas present.
   What is the most likely diagnosis?

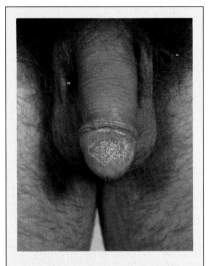

9. This man presented with a two-week history of pyrexia and arthralgia.
   (a) What physical sign is shown?
   (b) What is the likely underlying diagnosis?

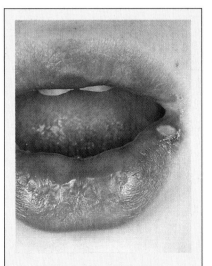

10. This lesion was associated with abdominal pain and tender joints. What is the probable underlying diagnosis?

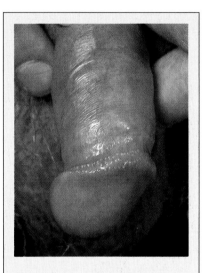

11. This man was worried about the appearance of his penis. What physical sign is demonstrated?

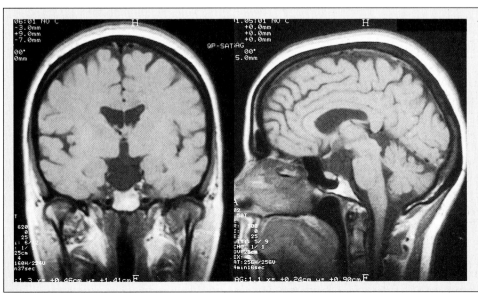

12. This scan is from a 54-year-old patient with intermittent profuse sweating attacks.
    (a) What is the abnormality?
    (b) What is the most likely underlying diagnosis?

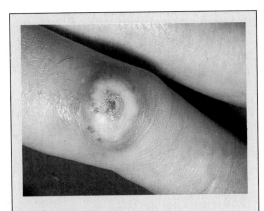

13. What is the diagnosis?

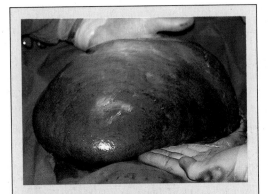

14. List two situations in which removal of this enlarged organ may be therapeutically indicated.

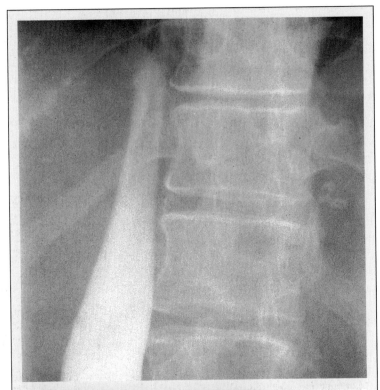

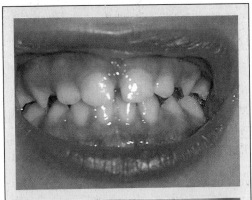

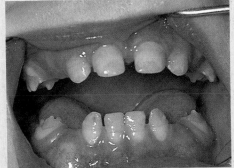

15. What is the most probable cause of this appearance?

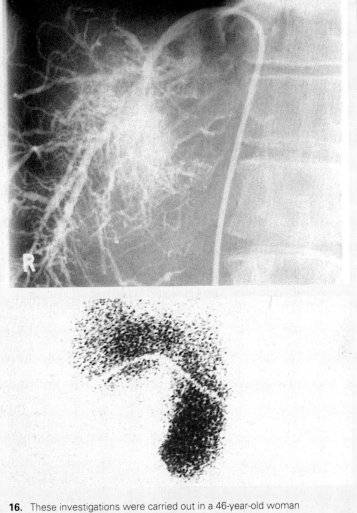

16. These investigations were carried out in a 46-year-old woman with tender hepatomegaly and recent onset of ascites.
   (a) What investigations are shown?
   (b) What is the diagnosis?

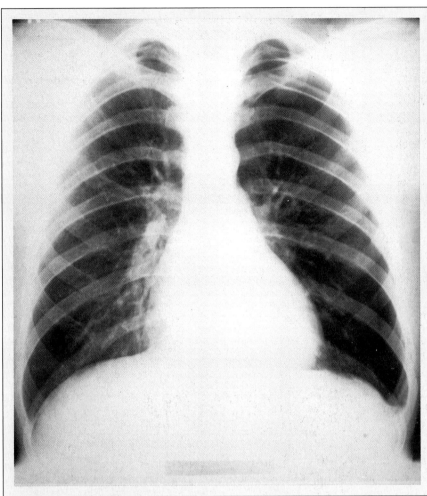

17. List two abnormalities on this chest radiograph.

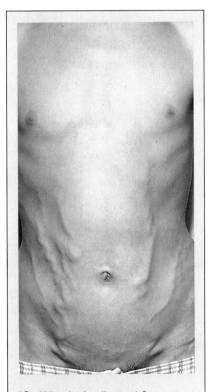

18. What is the diagnosis?

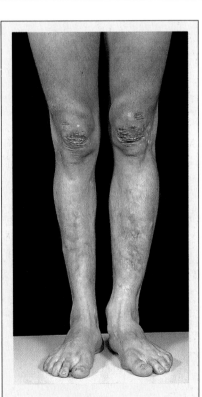

19. These are the legs of a man with recurrent anaemia.
What is the diagnosis?

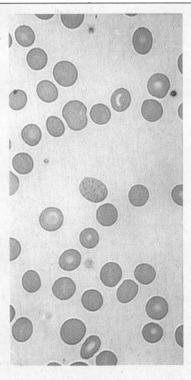

20. (a) What three abnormalities are shown on this blood film?
(b) Suggest a possible diagnosis.

Case Histories

CASE I

A 63-year-old woman was admitted to hospital following onset of severe diarrhoea and dehydration. She had been well until two years before, when degenerative arthritis of the hips was diagnosed. Her mobility became severely diminished, until she was confined to a bed and chair existence. Five months previously, she had experienced colicky abdominal pains associated with bouts of diarrhoea and constipation. The stools had become pellet-like. A barium enema examination showed severe diverticular disease. Ten days before admission, she began to complain of severe dysuria and frequency associated with a fever. Her GP prescribed a high fluid intake and antibiotic therapy. Her symptoms resolved, although weakness persisted. Three days before admission her abdominal pain recurred, this time associated with distension. She began to pass large volumes of liquid diarrhoea, green in colour. There was no blood, but some mucus was present.

On admission. the patient was clearly unwell but did not appear anaemic. Her skin was warm and dry with diminished turgor. Temperature 38.2°C, pulse 108/min regular; blood pressure 120/70mmHg lying, 100/60mmHg standing. Some ecchymoses were noted over the lower limbs. Cardiac auscultation revealed a grade II systolic ejection murmur at the left sternal border. The abdomen was distended and tympanitic, with diminished sounds. There was tenderness on deep palpation throughout the abdomen, but most markedly in the lower quadrants. There was no guarding or rebound tenderness. Liver, spleen and kidneys were not palpable. Rectal examination was normal.

Investigations

HAEMATOLOGY
Hb: 10.5g/dl (10.5g/100ml); PCV: 0.31 (31%); WBC: 29.4 × 10⁹/l (29,400/mm³); Neutrophils: 75%; Band forms: 18%; Lymphocytes: 5%; Monocytes: 2%; Platelets: 565 × 10⁹/l (565,000/mm³).

BIOCHEMISTRY
Sodium: 132mmol/l (132mEq/l); Potassium: 3.1mmol/l (3.1mEq/l); Chloride: 99mmol/l (99mEq/l); Bicarbonate: 18mmol/l (18mEq/l); Albumin: 24g/l (2.4g/100ml); Serum glutamic oxaloacetic transaminase (SGOT): 44iu/l; Alkaline phosphatase: 112iu/l (14.5KAU/100ml); Calcium: 2.1mmol/l (8.23mg/100ml); Urea: 14mmol/l (85mg/100ml); Creatinine: 130μmol/l (1.47mg/100ml); Urinanalysis: normal.

RADIOLOGY
Abdominal film: moderate gaseous distension of the stomach, diffuse dilatation of the small bowel loops and focal distension of the transverse and ascending portions of the colon, with prominent haustral folds. The ascending colon has a thumb-print pattern.

1. List two essential investigations.

2. What is the most likely diagnosis?

3. Suggest a second possible diagnosis.

CASE II

A 17-year-old girl was admitted to hospital because of drowsiness, headache, and some vomiting. Although her parents were Pakistani in origin, she herself was born in Britain. She was a vegan (strictly vegetarian), like her parents, and had always been in good health until three days before admission, when she developed a sudden onset of headache and dizziness. Shortly afterwards, she was incontinent of urine and developed a mild pyrexia. The GP requested admission.

On examination, she was drowsy, with a temperature of 37.6°C and mild neck stiffness. There was no photophobia. Pulse 90/min regular, blood pressure 140/90mmHg. Examination of the cardiovascular system revealed a normal jugular venous pulse and normally located apex beat, but auscultation revealed an ejection systolic murmur and a soft mid diastolic murmur at the apex. There were no splinter haemorrhages or splenomegaly, and the patient did not appear anaemic. In the central nervous system, she appeared to have a global dysphasia with weakness of the lower part of the right face. Tone was increased on the right with brisk reflexes, and the right plantar reflex was extensor. The rest of the clinical examination was normal.

Investigations

HAEMATOLOGY
Hb: 13.4g/dl (13.4 g/100ml); MCV: 81fl (81μm³); WBC: 7.4 × 10⁹/l (7,400/mm³); Neutrophils: 68%; Lymphocytes: 24%; Platelets: 280 × 10⁹/l (280,000/mm³); ESR: 62mm/h.

BIOCHEMISTRY & RADIOLOGY
Urea: 5.4mmol/l (33mg/100ml); Bilirubin: 14μmol/l (0.8mg/100ml); Alkaline phosphatase: 106iu/l (14KAU/100ml); Total protein: 68g/l (6.8g/100ml); Albumin: 33g/l (3.3g/100ml); Calcium: 2.4mmol/l (9.4mg/100ml); Phosphate: 0.96mmol/l (3.08mg/100ml); SGOT: 27iu/l; Urinanalysis: normal; CSF examination: blood-stained cerebrospinal fluid; Opening pressure: 180mmH₂O; RCC: 112 × 10⁹/l; WBC: 7 × 10⁶/l; Protein: 1g/l; Glucose: 4.8mmol/l (simultaneous blood glucose: 5.8mmol/l); Gram stain: no organisms seen; CXR: normal cardiac contour, lung fields clear; ECG: sinus rhythm normal QRS axis, no repolarisation abnormalities.

1. List four investigations which would be diagnostically helpful.

2. Suggest two possible diagnoses.

CASE III

A 43-year-old Indian woman presented with a six month history of discomfort and swelling in several fingers, her wrists, knees and feet. For four months she had suffered from recurrent painless blistering lesions on the extensor surface of the fingers and the palms in the region of the metacarpophalangeal joints. Each lesion would subsequently disappear within a few days. Four weeks prior to admission she had complained of a macular scaly rash on the back of her hands and the extensor surface of the arms, legs and feet, which resembled psoriasis. In the past she had been well and had lived in England for fifteen years, except for a four month visit to South India one year before presentation. There was a family history of osteoarthritis.

On examination, apart from the skin lesions and the changes in her joints, the patient was well-looking, with no lymphadenopathy. Pulse 70/min regular, blood pressure 130/90mmHg. The lungs were clear and heart sounds normal. All pulses were present, and dorsalis pedis pulses were bounding. Her peripheries were warm. Examination of the central nervous system revealed some alteration to pinprick sensation in both hands and feet. There was small muscle wasting in the hands. On her trunk there was a non-tender, oval, indurated area with well-defined margins.

Investigations

Hb: 13g/dl (13g/100ml); WBC: $6.9 \times 10^9/1$ (6,900/mm³); ESR: 12mm/h; Urea and electrolytes: normal; Liver function tests: normal; Uric acid estimation: 0.5mmol/l (5.0mg/100ml); Latex rheumatoid factor: negative; Antinuclear antibody: negative; Immunoelectrophoresis: slight rise in IgG; X-ray of the hands and wrists: periarticular osteoporosis present, and small erosions noted in the heads of the first metacarpal and second metatarsal bones.

1. List three investigations which would be useful.

2. What is the most likely diagnosis?

CASE IV

A 68-year-old retired nursing sister presented to her GP complaining of tiredness and generalised malaise. She was found to be anaemic clinically, and was referred to Outpatients. She had been unwell until nine months previously, when she began to complain of aches and pains in the limbs. On a number of occasions she had taken her own temperature and found it to be slightly raised. Recently, she complained of lack of energy, and even the simplest tasks would exhaust her. On specific enquiry, there was no history of blood loss or gastrointestinal symptoms, but she had lost 5kg in weight over three months.

On examination, the patient looked pale, and had a temperature of 37.4°C. She had clearly lost some weight. Blood pressure was 165/95mmHg. Cardiac auscultation revealed an ejection systolic murmur, which had a musical quality and was best audible at the left sternal edge. It did not radiate into the neck. The lungs were clear. No abnormality was detected on abdominal examination.

Investigations

Hb: 8.4g/dl (8.4g/100ml); WBC: $8.4 \times 10^9/l$ (8,400/mm³); Normocytic normochromic film; ESR: 84mm/h; Urea and electrolytes: normal; Liver function tests: normal; Antinuclear factor: negative; Rheumatoid factor: negative; CXR: some apical calcifications suggestive of old tubercle; Barium meal and abdominal ultrasound: negative; Faecal occult blood: negative; Urinanalysis: normal.

1. List three investigations which would be of greatest help in establishing a diagnosis.

2. Suggest three possible diagnoses.

CASE V

A 58-year-old right-handed cab driver was admitted to hospital for investigation of progressive right-sided weakness. He had been well until four weeks before when, while getting ready for work, he developed sudden onset of weakness involving the right hand and arm lasting about half an hour, with complete recovery. His GP diagnosed migraine, but the symptoms recurred a week later involving the same arm; on this occasion, recovery did not take place until 24 hours later. One week later, his right arm once again became weak, but this time weakness of the right wrist remained, which improved slightly, without full recovery. One week prior to admission, he developed facial weakness on the right side accompanied with a sensation of numbness, and two days later, on three consecutive occasions, there was loss of speech. During this time he felt confused, and in one of these episodes he seemed unable to see on his right side. There had been no loss of consciousness. In his medical history, apart from occasional migraines which he had suffered over 40 years, he had been healthy. Systemic enquiry was unremarkable.

On examination he was a cheerful, well-looking man with facial asymmetry and weakness of the lower right half of the face. Pulse 70/min regular, blood pressure 200/100mmHg with normal heart sounds. No carotid bruits were heard. Chest and abdominal examinations were normal. On detailed neurological examination, apart from the facial asymmetry, the cranial nerves were intact. There was, however, mild loss of sensation on the right side of the face. Tone was normal in both upper and lower limbs, but power was weak in a pyramidal distribution in the right arm and particularly distally. There was no pin-prick sensation on the dorsum of the right hand and fingers, but the thumb was spared. Joint positional sense was absent in the right hand. There was mild non-fluent dysphasia. Repetition was normal, with mild acalculia. He read slowly but accurately.

Investigations

HAEMATOLOGY
Hb: 15g/dl (15g/100ml); PCV: 0.44 (44%); WBC: $13.7 \times 10^9/l$ (13,700/mm³); Neutrophils: 62%; Platelets: $325 \times 10^9/l$ (325,000/mm³); ESR: 6mm/h.

BIOCHEMISTRY & RADIOLOGY
Urea: 4.8mmol/l (29mg/100ml); Creatinine: 0.10mmol/l (1.13mg/100ml); Sodium: 140mmol/l (140mEq/l); Chloride: 106mmol/l (106mEq/l); Bicarbonate: 24mmol/l (24mEq/l); Bilirubin: 17μmol/l (1mg/100ml); Alkaline phosphatase: 96iu/l (12KAU/100ml); Total protein: 74g/l (7.4g/100ml); Albumin: 44g/l (4.4g/100ml); Calcium: 2.33mmol/l (9.13mg/100ml); Phosphate: 1.25mmol/l (4.52mg/100ml); SGOT: 24iu/l; Fasting blood sugar: 4.4mmol/l (80mg/100ml); Urinanalysis: normal; CXR: normal; ECG: Sinus rhythm, normal QRS complexes, left axis deviation.

1. What two investigations are urgently indicated?

2. What is the most likely diagnosis?

Data Interpretations

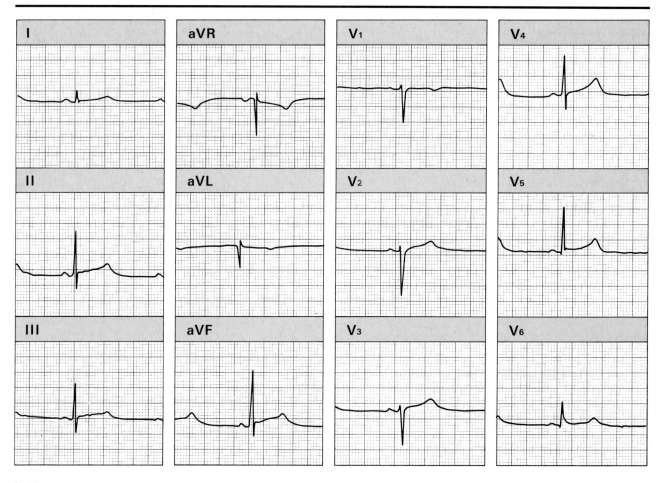

1. List three situations in which this electrocardiographic abnormality may be found.

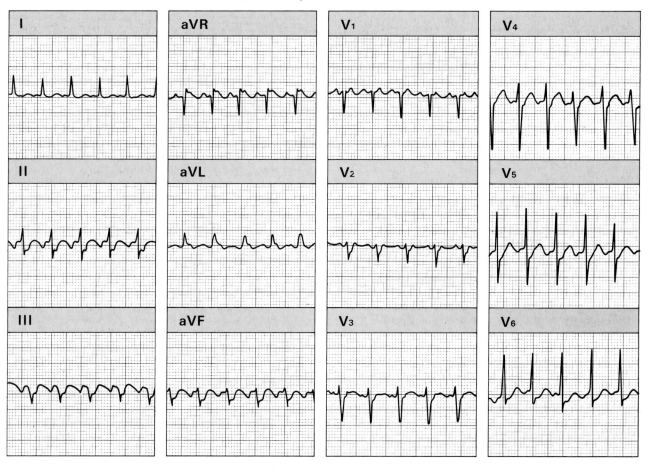

2. List two abnormalities on this electrocardiogram.

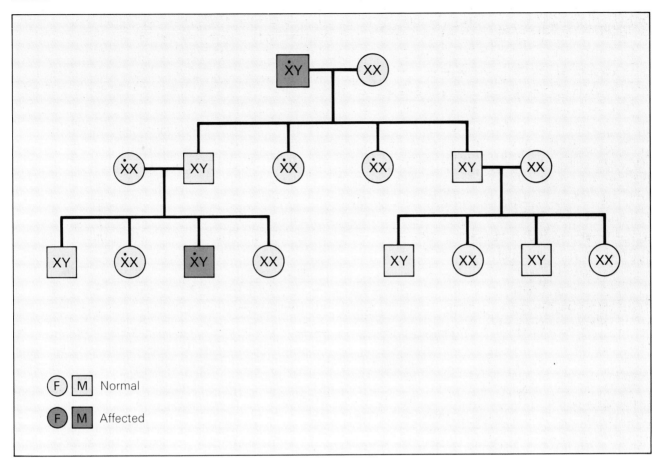

F M Normal

F M Affected

3. **(a)** What mode of transmission is demonstrated? **(b)** Give two examples.

4. A 44-year-old schizophrenic was admitted following a convulsion.
Sodium: 116mmol/l (116mEq/l); Plasma osmolality: 244mOsm/kg; Urinary specific gravity: 1.001.
What is the most likely diagnosis?

5. A 62-year-old man is under investigation for weight loss and a high ESR.
Sodium: 139mmol/l (139mEq/l); Potassium: 3.6mmol/l (3.6mEq/l); Bicarbonate: 24mmol/l (24mEq/l); Chloride: 116mmol/l (116mEq/l); Lactate: 1mmol/l.
(a) What abnormality is shown?
(b) Give a possible cause.

6. A 25-year-old woman in the first trimester of pregnancy gives a 48 hour history of a generalised macular rash.
Rubella CFT: 1/64; Rubella IgM: negative.
(a) What conclusions can be drawn from these results?
(b) What advice should be given to her?

7. Following a visit to Eastern Europe, a 23-year-old female student complains of loose stools, crampy abdominal pain and a 6kg weight loss.
Hb: 10.9g/dl (10.9g/100ml); MCV: 79fl (79μm^3); Albumin: 31g/l; Film: dimorphic.
(a) Give three investigations which would assist in establishing the underlying diagnosis.
(b) Suggest one possible diagnosis.

8. A 22-year-old girl presents with gross acanthosis nigricans and persistent glycosuria. As part of her investigations, an insulin tolerance test is carried out.

Time (min)	Glucose (mmol/l)
0 insulin 0.15U/kg	9.4
15	7.4
30 insulin 0.3U/kg	7.1
45	4.5
60	3.8
75	3.5
90	5.9
120	8.5

What inferences can be drawn from these findings?

9. After admission for chest pain and pyrexia a 56-year-old woman with known breast cancer has the following blood count
Hb: 11.4g/dl (11.4g/100ml); MCV: 87fl (87μm^3); WBC: 23 × 10^9/l (23,000/mm^3); Neutrophils: 88%; Lymphocytes: 6%; Metamyelocytes: 4%; Myelocytes: 2%; Promyelocytes: 1%; Platelets: 80 × 10^9/l (80,000/mm^3).
(a) What abnormality is present?
(b) Suggest three essential investigations.

10. A 21-year-old male is investigated for a short history of lethargy and anorexia. On examination, a faint maculopapular rash is found on the trunk and the extremities.
Hb: 13.4g/dl (13.4g/100ml); PCV: 0.44 (34%); MCV: 94fl (94μm^3); WBC: 14.4 × 10^9/l (14,400/mm^3); Neutrophils: 38%; Lymphocytes: 19%; Reactive lymphocytes: 20%; Platelets: 210 × 10^9/l (210,000/mm^3); Film: agglutination ++, polychromasia ++.
(a) Suggest two possible diagnoses.
(b) Suggest four diagnostically helpful investigations.

Answers

1. Neuropathic ulcer ★★★★
   Ischaemic ulcer 0
   This is a typical site for a neuropathic ulcer. Underlying causes include:
   Diabetes mellitus;
   Leprosy;
   Syphilis (tabes dorsalis);
   Congenital absence of pain.
   Neuropathic (or neurotrophic) ulcers on the feet are seen, particularly on the pressure bearing areas, under the heads of the metatarsals and on the heel.

2. Lead poisoning ★★★★
   Gingival hyperplasia (phenytoin-related folic acid deficiency) ★
   Lead sulphide has been deposited along the gingival margin of some teeth, producing the pathognomonic blue-black lead line.

3. (a) Central retinal vein occlusion ★★★★
       Papilloedema ★★★★
   (b) Paraproteinaemia ★★★★
       Systemic lupus erythematosus ★★★★
       Nephrotic syndrome ★★★★
       Hyperlipidaemia ★★★★
   All retinal veins are pathologically engorged with blood and extremely tortuous, and the retina is covered with haemorrhages. Macular oedema and soft exudates may be present. Central retinal vein occlusion has an increased incidence in diabetes mellitus, collagen vascular diseases, hypertension, and hyperviscocity syndromes. Fasting lipids, plasma proteins, a glucose tolerance test and Hb estimation are warranted investigations.

4. Right ulnar nerve lesion ★★★★ Froments Sign.
   Weak right first interossei ★★
   There is weakness of the right first interosseous, due to an ulnar nerve lesion. Function of the thumb is profoundly affected by ulnar nerve loss.

5. Prolactinoma ★★★★
   Hyperprolactinaemia ★★★★
   Primary hypothyroidism ★★★★
   Dopamine antagonists ★★★★
   Hyperprolactinaemia (with galactorrhoea) found in association with primary hypothyroidism is thought to be in part due to the high hypothalamo-hypophyseal portal venous levels of TRH, which is thought to be a physiological stimulator of prolactin (and of course TSH) secretion.

6. Impetigo contagiosum ★★★★
   Contact dermatitis 0
   Eczema 0
   Exfoliative dermatitis 0
   This is a superficial primary pyoderma caused by either group A beta haemolytic streptococci, or a staphylococcus of bacteriophage type 71. Lesions begin as macules and progress to vesicles and bullae which rupture, releasing a cloudy yellow fluid that forms crusts; when removed, a weeping denuded area is revealed.

7. (a) Sarcoidosis ★★★★
   (b) Anterior and posterior uveitis ★★★★
       Keratoconjunctivitis ★★★★
       Scleral plaques ★★★★
       Retinal vasculitis ★★★★
       Lacrimal gland enlargement ★★★★
       Papilloedema ★★★★
       Secondary glaucoma ★★★★
       Cataract formation ★★★★
       Corneal band opacities ★★★★

In addition to the above, there are several well defined ocular syndromes associated with sarcoidosis:
Heerfordt's or Waldenström's syndrome (uveitis, parotid enlargement, fever, seventh nerve palsy); Löfgren's syndrome (erythema nodosum, bilateral hilar lymphadenopathy, iritis); Sjögren-like syndrome with keratoconjunctivitis.
Cutaneous manifestations of sarcoidosis include:
Erythema nodosum; Lupus pernio; Maculopapular rashes; Plaques; Subcutaneous nodules.

8. Leprosy ★★★★
   Syphilis 0
   Lepromatous leprosy is characterized by widespread skin lesions. Patients with tuberculoid leprosy have fewer skin lesions, but are also subject to peripheral nerve damage. Occasionally, skin lesions are absent altogether; this pure neural leprosy represents a mono-neuritis multiplex involving one or more nerves of predilection, which are characteristically thickened. The resulting anaesthesia may lead to neuroarthropathic features and deformity (shown here).

9. (a) Balanitis circinata ★★★★
       Penile psoriasis ★★
       Erythema multiforme ★
   (b) Reiter's syndrome ★★★★
   Penile lesions occur in 25% of patients with Reiter's syndrome, their morphology on the glans depending on the presence or absence of a foreskin. In the uncircumcised man, a shallow, red, moist erosion develops, which coalesces. In the circumcised man, the erosions quickly become covered by a mixture of crust and scale, evolving into the typical keratoderma appearance.

10. Inflammatory bowel disease ★★★★
    Behçet's disease ★★★★
    Reiter's syndrome ★
    Vasculitis ★
    This was an aphthous ulcer in a patient with Crohn's disease.

11. Pearly penile papules ★★★★
    Hairy penis ★★★★
    Penile pupillae ★★★★
    Penile warts 0
    Reassurance is called for. Penile pupillae are a normal finding which occurs between the ages of 20–50, and are best considered as angiofibromas. An incidence of 10% has been recorded.

12. (a) A mass in the suprasellar region, extending into the interpeduncular fossa abutting the upper pontine region. It seems to be extending into the third ventricle ★★★★
    (b) Arachnoid cyst ★★★★
    Swellings or masses around this part of the brain may precipitate a diencephalic syndrome consisting of intermittent episodes of severe sweating with hypothermia.

13. Orf ★★★★
    (syn.: erythema contagiosum, contagious pustular dermatitis)
    This is a disease widespread in sheep, affecting mainly young lambs. Human lesions are caused by direct innoculation of infected material, and are seen in shepherds, veterinary surgeons and farmers' wives who bottle-feed lambs. After an incubation period of five to six days, a small, firm, reddish blue papule forms, enlarging into a flat-topped haemorrhagic pustule or bulla, often crusted in its umbilicated centre. In the fully developed lesion, the central crust is surrounded by the characteristic greyish-white ring, encircled by a zone of erythema. Spontaneous recovery occurs within three to five weeks.

14. Myelofibrosis ★★★★
    Gaucher's disease ★★★★

Felty's syndrome ★★★★
This is a case of massive splenomegaly. Other indications for splenectomy include:
Haemolytic anaemia in which splenic sequestration and destruction can be ascertained;
Acute splenic vascular accidents, or if there is discomfort or threat of rupture in massive splenomegaly from any cause;
Immunologically mediated thrombocytopenia;
Staging in Hodgkin's disease;
Severe hypersplenism due to infiltrative or hyperplastic splenomegaly.

15. Tetracycline staining of teeth ★★★★
This antimicrobial agent can cause staining and hypoplasia of dental enamel, as well as disturbed bone growth in neonates and young children.

16. (a) Hepatic venogram showing filling defects in the common hepatic vein and collateral vessel formation ★★★★
Inferior vena cavogram showing an obstruction to the flow of contrast at the level of D.11 ★★★★
Technetium (^{99m}Tc) scan of liver/spleen showing increased activity in the caudate lobe with reduced uptake in the rest of the liver ★★★★
(b) Budd–Chiari syndrome ★★★★

17. Small left pneumothorax ★★★★
Right hilar lymph node calcification ★★★★
Hilar lymph node calcification is most commonly seen with old tuberculosis. Other causes of 'eggshell' calcification of hilar lymph nodes include silicosis, sarcoidosis, lymphoma following radiotherapy, and coal miner's pneumoconiosis.

18. Inferior vena caval obstruction ★★★★
Caput medusae 0
There is an extensive collateral circulation involving the inferior epigastric veins. The flow of blood is upward from the groin.

19. Ehlers-Danlos syndrome ★★★★
Papyraceous scars on knees ★★★★
Cutis laxa ★★
This condition results from a generalised defect of connective tissue, the inheritance of which is usually determined by an autosomal dominant gene. The essential defect is a quantitative deficiency of collagen. The characteristic features are fragility of the skin and blood vessels, hyperelasticity of the skin and joint hyperextensibility. Trivial lacerations of the skin result in gaping wounds which heal slowly. These leave broad papyraceous scars in which blue-grey spongy tumours (molluscoid pseudotumours) may form. Trauma over the shins, knees (shown here) and elbows produces cigarette paper-thin scars.

20. (a) Anisocytosis ★★★★
Oval macrocytes ★★★★
Thrombocytopenia ★★★★
(b) Megaloblastic anaemia due to B12 or folate deficiency ★★★★
Primary laboratory findings in B12 deficiency include oval macrocytes, leukopenia, thrombocytopenia and a megaloblastic marrow. In temporal sequence in evolving folic acid deficiency, first hypersegmented neutrophils are found, then oval macrocytes and finally anaemia.

ANSWERS TO CASE HISTORIES

Case I

1. Sigmoidoscopy with rectal biopsy ★★★★
Isolation of clostridium difficile toxin from stool ★★★★
Blood cultures ★★★★
Abdominal ultrasound ★

2. Antibiotic-related diarrhoea ★★★★
Pseudomembranous enterocolitis (probably secondary to ampicillin therapy) ★★★★

3. Staphylococcal enterocolitis ★★★★
Toxic dilatation of the colon (secondary to ulcerative colitis) ★★★★
Ischaemic colitis ★
Pseudomembranous enterocolitis is an inflammatory condition affecting small and large bowel. The disease is usually seen in patients with serious underlying illness, such as shock or ischaemia of the intestine. Clostridium difficile toxin is thought to be the causative agent. The involved bowel is covered with yellowish-green membranous plaques which become confluent.

Case II

1. Blood cultures ★★★★
Cardiac echocardiogram ★★★★
Contast-enhanced CT scan of head ★★★★
Technetium pertechnate (^{99m}Tc) brain scan ★★
VDRL TPHA ★
ANF ★
Left carotid arteriogram 0

2. Left atrial myxoma with cerebral infarct ★★★★
SBE with septic embolus ★★★★
Herpes simplex encephalitis ★★
Cerebral infarct/haemorrhage ★★
Mitral stenosis with embolus ★
Subarachnoid haemorrhage ★
Composition of CSF after CVA (intracranial bleeding):
Soon after bleeding: White cell count is commensurate with amount of bleeding, i.e. 1 white cell for 1000 red cells.
>12 hours after bleeding: The WCC is increased, due to the inflammatory reaction in the meninges, and may reach levels of 500×10^6/l. Early in the course of the inflammatory response, polymorphs predominate. Later on, lymphocytes are found. An exudate protein response accompanies intracranial haemorrhage, often with levels >lg/l. With acute bleeding for each 10,000 red cells in the CSF, the protein rises to 0.15g/l.

Case III

1. Skin biopsy of the rash on feet and trunk ★★★★
Electromyography ★★★★
Nerve biopsy ★★★★
Chest X-ray ★★★★

2. Tuberculoid leprosy ★★★★
SLE ★
Lupus vulgaris 0
Yaws 0
In tuberculoid leprosy, skin lesions are single or few and are sharply demarcated. Neurological involvement is relatively pronounced, and peripheral nerves are often palpable. There may be severe neuritic pain, and muscle atrophy especially of the small muscles of the hand. The histological picture consists of lymphocytes, epithelioid cells and giant cells. Bacilli are few; the lepromin reaction is usually positive.

Case IV

1. EMU and gastric washings for AFB ★★★★
Bone marrow examination and culture for AFB ★★★★
Temporal artery biopsy ★★★★
Serum electrophoresis ★★
Reticulocyte count ★
B12 and folate estimations ★
Echocardiogram ★
Bone marrow examination for iron stones ★
IVU ★

Answers

2. Occult malignancy ★★★★
   Giant cell arteritis ★★★★
   Polymyalgia rheumatica ★★★★
   Tuberculosis ★★
   Subacute bacterial endocarditis ★★
   Polymyositis ★
   Mantoux test ★

Case V

1. Contrast enhanced CT scan ★★★★
   Carotid angiogram ★★★★
   Digital substraction scan ★★
   Echocardiogram ★★
   VDRL TPHA ★★
   24 hour ECG ★★
   Doppler study of the carotids ★
   CSF examination 0

2. A stroke in evolution, probably involving the left middle cerebral
   territory ★★★★
   Left hemispheric tumour ★★
   Left subdural haematoma ★
   Meningioma ★
   Stroke in evolution is characterised by the development of step-
   like paralysis and sensory impairment over a number of hours or
   days. The territory involved here is the left middle cerebral artery.
   Gradual infarction of this territory causes damage to the lateral
   part of the hemisphere, producing a variable degree of
   contralateral paresis and sensory loss. This involves mainly the
   face, the upper limbs (particularly the hands), and frequently
   causes a right homonymous visual field loss. In the absence of a
   contraindication, this patient should be anticoagulated forthwith.

ANSWERS TO DATA INTERPRETATIONS

1. Drug-induced QT interval prolongation ★★★★
   Hypocalcaemia ★★★★
   Hypomagnesaemia ★★★★
   Congenital long QT syndrome ★★★★
   Romano-Ward syndrome ★★★★
   Jervell-Lange-Nielsen syndrome ★★★★
   There is prolongation of the QT interval, and a sinus bradycardia.
   Quinidine, procainamide and disopyramide may prolong the QT
   interval. Other drugs include prenylamine and phenothiazines, as
   well as tricyclic antidepressants.

2. Atrial flutter with 2:1 block ★★★★
   Inferior subendocardial ischaemia ★★★★
   Poor 'R' wave progression V1–V4 ★★★★

3. (a) X-linked recessive ★★★★
   (b) Red-green colour blindness ★★★★
       Haemophilia A ★★★★

4. Water intoxication ★★★★
   Inappropriate ADH secretion 0
   This situation arose because the patient consumed more water
   than can be excreted by the normal kidney (i.e. 1–1.2l/h). The
   resulting expansion of extracellular volume leads to
   hyponatraemia and renal wasting of sodium. Chronic ingestion of
   large volumes of water impairs the renal concentrating
   mechanism, making the distinction between primary polydipsia
   and true diabetes insipidus more difficult, although a simple
   water deprivation test will usually differentiate between the two.

5. (a) Absence of anion gap ★★★★
       Hyperchloraemia ★★
   (b) Paraproteinaemia ★★★★
       Hypermagnesaemia, hypoalbuminaemia and bromide intake will
       also produce this type of abnormality. In paraproteinaemia the
       proteins have a high cationic charge which will retain chloride.

6. (a) Rubella immunity present ★★★★
   (b) Check titres again in two weeks, but the patient should be
       reassured ★★★★

7. (a) Stool microscopy for cysts ★★★★
       Duodenal aspirate for trophozoites ★★★★
       Barium studies to exclude Crohn's disease ★★★★
       Jejunal biopsy ★★★★
       Fe/TIBC determination ★★★★
       Folate/B12 estimation ★★
       Immunoglobulin electrophoresis ★
   (b) Giardiasis with malabsorption ★★★★
       Crohn's disease ★★
   Giardiasis is one cause of steatorrhea. There is an association
   between symptomatic giardiasis and hypogammaglobulinaemia.
   Active infection may be associated with villous flattening,
   abnormal fat balance and D-xylose tests. Epigastric pain
   resembling a peptic ulcer may be a major symptom.

8. Severe insulin resistance ★★★★
   This type of insulin-resistant diabetes mellitus, associated with
   acanthosis nigricans, is found (rarely) in young females. It is
   related to the presence of an antibody to the insulin receptor, in
   the same way as in the lipoatrophic diabetic. Other patients have
   a variant of this condition in association with other autoimmune
   diseases such as RLA and SLE.

9. (a) Leukaemoid reaction (secondary to neoplastic marrow
       infiltration) ★★★★
       Leucoerythroblastic anaemia 0
   (b) Bone marrow trephine to exclude infiltration ★★★★
       Bone scan ★★★★
       Chest X-ray to exclude infection ★★★★
       Blood cultures ★★★★
       LAP score (increased in leukaemoid reaction) ★★★★
   In leukaemoid reactions, the peripheral blood film resembles that
   of leukaemia, usually, but not invariably, in the context of a raised
   white cell count. Leukaemoid reactions may involve any of the
   white blood cells, and may be triggered by: Bacterial and viral
   infections; Allergy; Inflammatory disease; Poisoning, drugs;
   Malignancy; Physical and emotional stimuli; Haemolytic anaemia;
   Haemorrhage; Burns.

10. (a) Infectious mononucleosis ★★★★
        Cytomegalovirus (CMV) infection ★★★★
        Toxoplasma infection ★★★★
        Mycoplasma pneumoniae infection ★★
    (b) Monospot test ★★★★
        Viral titres for CMV ★★★★
        Urinary isolation of CMV ★★★★
        Paul Bunnell test ★★
        Direct Coombs' test ★★
        Bilirubin level/reticulocyte count ★★
        Liver function tests ★★
        Search for cold agglutinins ★★
        Mycoplasma titres ★★
        Sabin-Feldman dye test for toxoplasma infection ★★

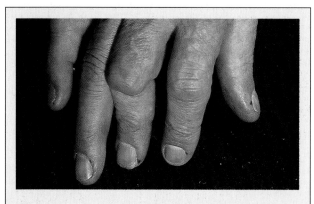

1. What is the most likely diagnosis?

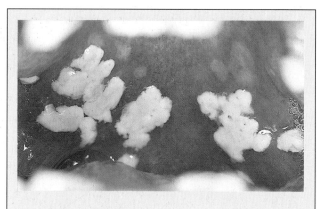

2. (a) What is the diagnosis?
   (b) Give three associations.

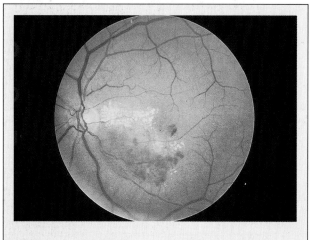

3. What is the diagnosis?

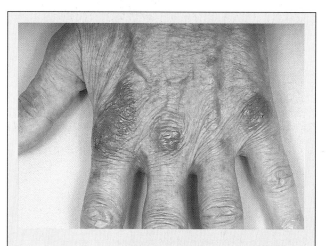

4. What is the most likely cause of this painless eruption?

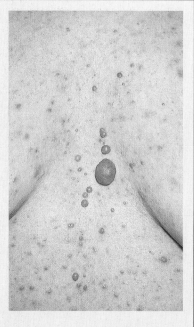

5. What is the diagnosis?

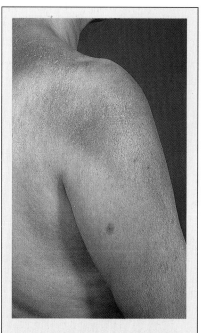

6. This pigmented lesion had been present for several months in a patient under investigation for heavy proteinuria.
   Suggest a likely diagnosis.

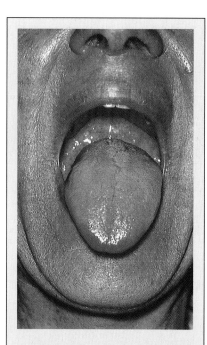

7. This man presented with recurrent episodes of amaurosis fugax. Splenomegaly was also present. Suggest a likely underlying diagnosis.

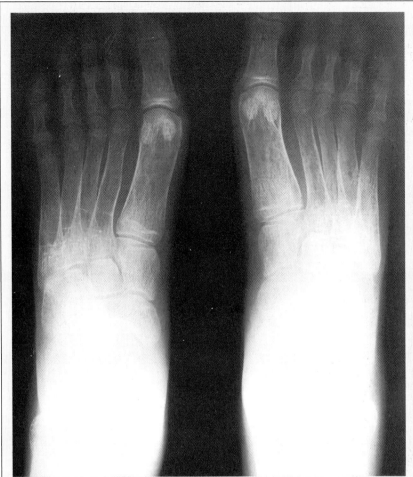 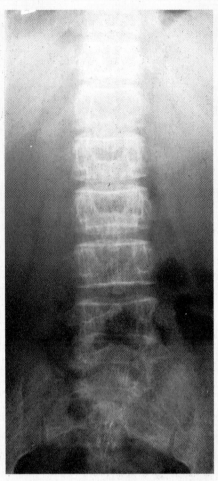

8. These radiographs were from a 21-year-old patient with a haemoglobin of 5.3g/dl and an MCV of 60 fl. What is the probable diagnosis?

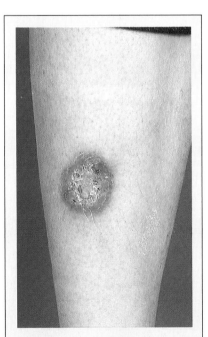

9. This painless lesion appeared over a number of weeks over the skin of a 65-year-old woman. What is the likely diagnosis?

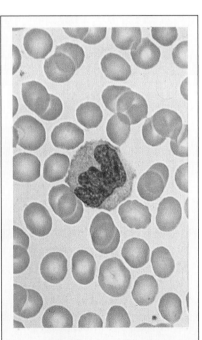

10. What diagnosis can be inferred from this bone marrow examination?

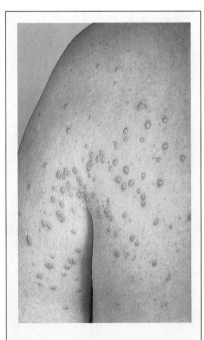

11. What is the most likely diagnosis?

Slide Interpretations

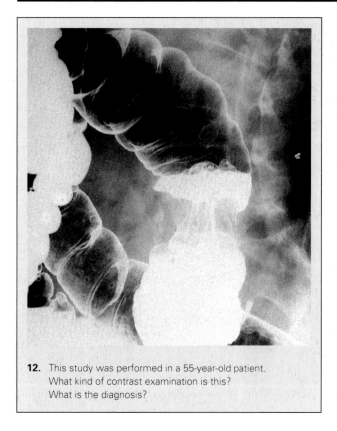

12. This study was performed in a 55-year-old patient.
    What kind of contrast examination is this?
    What is the diagnosis?

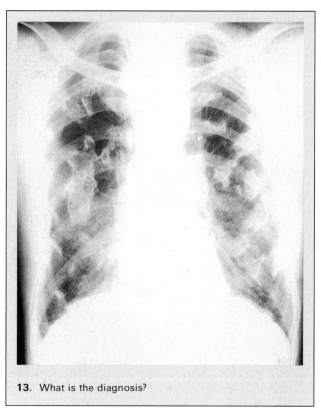

13. What is the diagnosis?

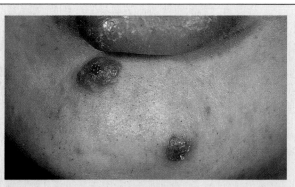

14. These lesions were found in a female patient with a
    chronic cough and dyspnoea.
    What is the most probable diagnosis?

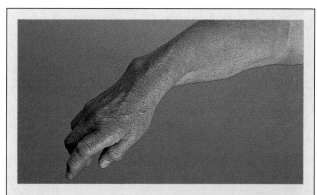

15. This patient complained of long-standing pain in her
    forearm.
    What is the diagnosis?

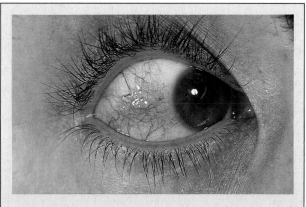

16. This is the eye of a girl under treatment for a chronic
    abdominal ailment.
    What is the diagnosis?

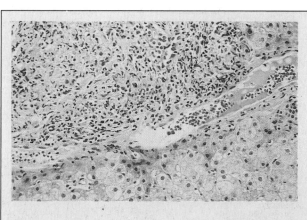

17. This is a liver biopsy specimen stained with H&E.
    What is the diagnosis?

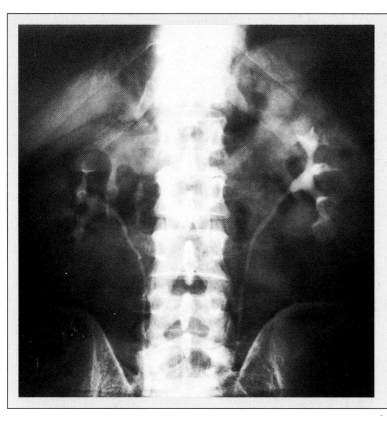

18. This contrast radiograph is from a patient under investigation for renal colic. What is the diagnosis?

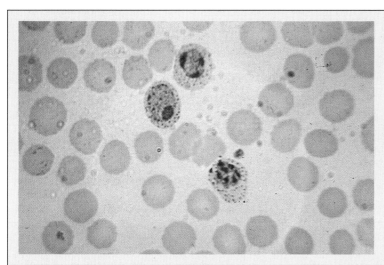

19. What is the diagnosis?

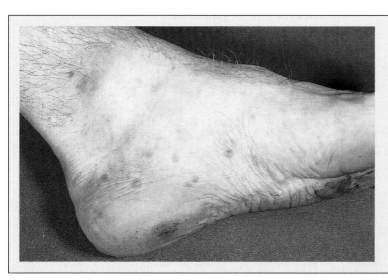

20. Give a possible cause for these painless lesions.

Case Studies

CASE I

A 51-year-old Caucasian housewife, residing in South London, presented with a three-month history of progressive malaise, lethargy and fevers, and a weight loss of 10kg. Five months previously, she had visited Portugal for a two-week holiday, after which she had suffered an episode of non-bloody diarrhoea which lasted twelve days. Thereafter her bowel habit returned to normal. However, she continued to feel unwell, and complained of feeling hot and shivery once or twice a week. In her past medical history, she had had epigastric pain diagnosed as a duodenal ulcer, which was successfully treated with a course of cimetidine. Her menses had always been somewhat irregular, and she had reached the menopause at the age of 43.

On examination, she was pale and had a swinging pyrexia sometimes reaching 39.6°C. There was no lymphadenopathy noted, and examination of the heart and lungs was unremarkable. Blood pressure was 150/95mmHg. Examination of the abdomen revealed a mass arising from the left hypochondrium which was dull to percussion and moved downwards with respiration. Rectal, vaginal and central nervous system examinations were unremarkable.

Investigations

Hb: 9.3g/dl (9.3g/100ml); MCV: 76fl (76μm^3);
WBC: 3.0 × 10^9/l (3,000/mm^3); Neutrophils: 62%;
Lymphocytes: 18%; Monocytes: 18%; Platelets: 102 × 10^9/l (102,000/mm^3); ESR: 79mm/h; Direct Coombs' test: weakly positive; Urea and electrolytes: normal; Liver function tests: normal; Rheumatoid factor: weakly positive; Urinanalysis: normal; CXR: normal.

1. List five investigations that you consider diagnostically useful.

2. Suggest two possible diagnoses.

CASE II

A 16-year-old boy was admitted for investigation of non-specific central chest pain and progressive exertional dyspnoea. He had been well in the past, with normal developmental milestones. However, from the age of 13 years he had been in constant trouble with the police for petty theft, and over the last year he had taken to glue sniffing. In his past medical history, he had had pneumonia in childhood, and six months before he had seen his GP because of two syncopal attacks for which no cause was found.

On examination, he was dyspnoeic at rest, with a pulse of 110/min regular and blood pressure 120/80mmHg. His weight was 58kg. The jugulovenous pulse was raised by 4cm and the apex beat was displaced to the left. Examination of the praecordium revealed biventricular enlargement. Cardiac auscultation revealed a gallop rhythm, with a loud pulmonary component of the second sound. All pulses were present and equal. Auscultation of the lungs revealed crackles from both mid zones to the bases. The liver was enlarged by 3cm and slightly tender. There was no other organomegaly, and no ascites. The rest of the clinical examination was unremarkable, except for mild ankle oedema.

Investigations

HAEMATOLOGY
Hb: 14.6g/dl (14.6g/100ml); PCV: 0.51 (51%); MCV: 84fl (84μm^3); WBC: 6.8 × 10^9/l (6,800/mm^3); Normal differential count; ESR: 28mm/h; Urea and electrolytes: normal; Alkaline phosphatase: 188iu/l (24.4KAU/100ml).

RADIOLOGY & SPECIAL INVESTIGATIONS
CXR: Cardiomegaly and Kerley B-lines in both lower lung fields; ECG: normal PR interval, intraventricular conduction abnormality in V$_1$–V$_6$ and aVL. T-wave inversion in lead I and aVL; Cardiac catheter data: Pulmonary artery pressure: 50/20mmHg; Pulmonary artery wedge pressure: 24mmHg; LVEDP: 22mmHg; Cardiac output: 5.6 l/min.

1. List three investigations which would be diagnostically useful.

2. Suggest two possible causes for his presentation.

CASE III

A 23-year-old secretary consulted her GP because, following a bout of flu, she had noticed that she was dragging her feet and that her legs felt heavy. On examination, the GP found little wrong and reassured her. Three days later, her left breast became uncomfortable and she noticed that running her hand over the lower half of the breast caused a most unpleasant sensation. Shortly afterwards, she developed an ache on the right from the groin to the knee, which she described feeling as if the flesh was being torn from the bones. This sensation seemed worse on coughing and straining. She was referred to her local neurological clinic as an urgent case, but on the day of admission she developed urinary urgency.

On examination, the patient was looking well and was neither anaemic nor clubbed. Her weight was 61kg, pulse 76/min regular, blood pressure 130/70mmHg. Examination of the heart and lungs was normal, as was examination of the cranial nerves. On further neurological testing, tone was found to be generally increased in the lower limbs, and there was bilateral weakness of the flexors. Some clonus could be elicited, particularly on the left. Abdominal jerks appeared absent, and extensor responses could be elicited bilaterally. On sensory testing, there appeared to be an area of altered sensation over the left breast, and diminution to pinprick and temperature sensation in the entire right leg extending to just below the level of the umbilicus. Joint positional sense was impaired in the left leg, but it was normal on the right. Abdominal examination was normal.

Investigations

Hb: 13.2g/dl (13.2g/100ml); MCV: 83fl (83μm^3); MCH 29pg (29$\mu\mu$g); WBC: 6.8 × 10^9/l (6,800/mm^3); Normal differential count; ESR: 23mm/h; Urea: 5.6mmol/l (34mg/100ml); Sodium: 139mmol/l (139mEq/l); Potassium: 4.6mmol/l (4.6mEq/l); Chloride: 98mmol/l (98mEq/l); Bicarbonate: 27mmol/l (27mEq/l); Urinanalysis: normal; CXR: heart size normal, lungs clear.

1. List two investigations which should be carried out as a matter of urgency.

2. Suggest one possible diagnosis.

CASE IV

A 71-year-old retired tailor was admitted to hospital because of periorbital swelling. He had been well until eight months previously, when he began to suffer from anorexia and some weight loss which totalled 7kg by the time of presentation. One morning, three months before, he woke up with swelling and pain around his right orbit. Over the ensuing 24 hours, he became unable to move his right eye in any direction of gaze, as any such attempt caused him pain. He was referred to a local ophthalmologist who diagnosed a periorbital cellulitis. ESR was 110mm/h. He was treated with a combination of amoxycillin, flucloxacillin and metronidazole. The swelling gradually subsided over the ensuing three weeks. The patient was quite well after his first course of antibiotics, and for the following two months he remained asymptomatic. Five days prior to admission, he woke up with pain and swelling in the left eye.

On admission, the orbital region was swollen and the conjunctiva was red. Eye movements seemed limited, but fundal examination was normal and visual acuity was not impaired. He was pyrexial at 37.8°C. Systemic examination revealed no abnormal signs in the heart, lungs or abdomen, and there was no lymphadenopathy. Examination of his legs, however, revealed large numbers of confluent, round, macular erythematous lesions, with pale areas in their centres. A purpuric lesion was present in the nailfold of his right large toe. In the calf, the superficial veins were tender and thrombosed.

Investigations

Hb: 9.8g/dl (9.8g/100ml); WBC: 13 × 10⁹/l (13,000/mm³); Neutrophils: 81%; Lymphocytes: 9%; Rouleaux: +++; ESR: 127mm/h; Reticulocytes: 2%; Normochromic normocytic film; Liver function tests: normal; Serum electrophoresis: raised α_2 globulin; Urinanalysis: normal; ECG: normal; CXR: normal.

1. List four investigations which would help in establishing the underlying diagnosis.

2. Suggest a likely diagnosis.

CASE V

A 25-year-old man, with known congenital cyanotic heart disease, was admitted with a ten-day history of headaches initially brought on by strenuous exercise, and more recently precipitated by even mild exercise. He had been cyanosed about four months after birth, and was diagnosed to be suffering from 'a hole in the heart'. Despite this, he had been remarkably well, and had had normal developmental milestones. He was prone to headaches and was receiving, every two to three months, a venesection which relieved his symptoms. Four weeks previously, he had decided to take a long vacation to the West Indies. It was upon his return from this otherwise uneventful holiday that the headache recommenced. However, until that time, its association with exercise had not been noted.

On examination, he was cyanosed, with obvious clubbing of the fingers. Pulse 98/min regular, blood pressure 130/90mmHg. His jugulovenous pulse was raised by 3cm, and the apex beat was not displaced. A left parasternal heave was noted. Cardiac auscultation revealed a pansystolic murmur, best heard on the left side of the sternum in the fourth intercostal space; the second sound was not split. The lungs were clear. There was nothing of note in the abdomen, and examination of the central nervous system was unremarkable. The fundi, in particular, were entirely normal. A pyrexia of 37.5°C was noted.

Investigations

Hb: 21.6g/dl (21.6g/100ml); RCC: 8.0 × 10⁹/l (8,000/mm³); MCV: 78fl (78μm³); WBC: 9.6 × 10⁹/l (9,600/mm³); Neutrophils: 80%; Lymphocytes: 15%; Platelets: 406 × 10⁹/l (406,000/mm³); ESR: 8mm/h; Urea and electrolytes: normal; Liver function tests: normal; CXR: lung fields clear, the cardiac contour slightly globular; ECG: sinus rhythm, tall peaked P-waves present, gross right axial deviation of the heart, evidence of right ventricular hypertrophy; Urinanalysis: normal.

1. List three essential investigations in this patient's management.

2. What is the most likely underlying diagnosis?

Data Interpretations

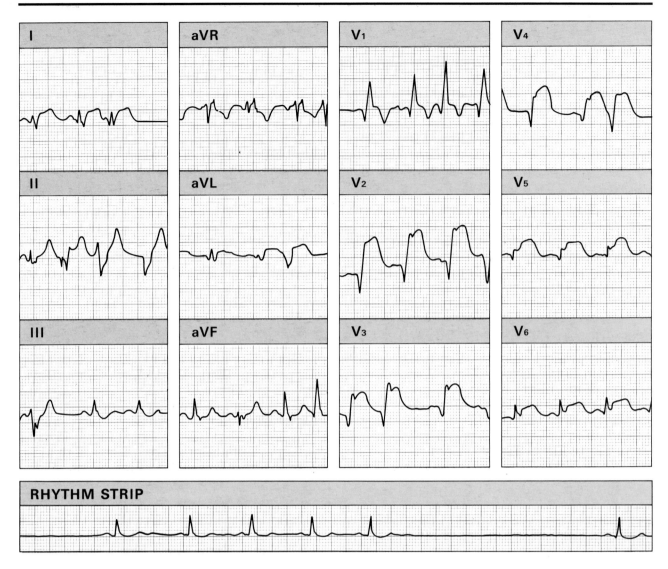

1. List three abnormalities in this electrocardiogram.

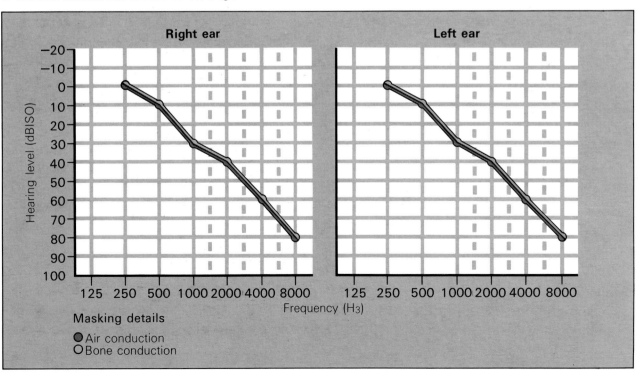

2. Suggest a likely cause for this audiometric appearance.

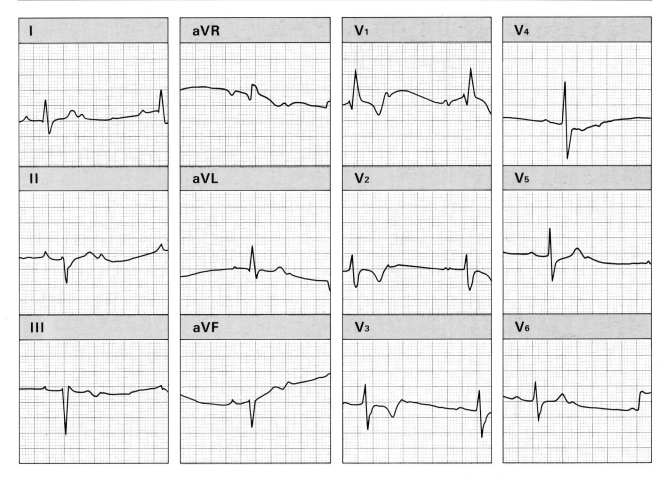

I	aVR	V1	V4
II	aVL	V2	V5
III	aVF	V3	V6

3. What abnormalities are present on this ECG?

4. A 7-year-old girl is investigated for cyanosis and short stature.
Hb: 21.4g/dl (21.4g/100ml); PaO2: 5.7kPa (43mmHg); PaCO2: 5.2kPa (39mmHg).
List two possible causes for the above findings.

5. Six days following a large myocardial infarction, a 54-year-old man develops purplish and painful discolouration of the nose and fingers of the right hand. On examination, there is bruising on the legs and trunk.
Hb: 11.7g/dl (11.7g/100ml); Platelets 25 × 10⁹/l (25,000/mm³); Polychromasia: ++; PT: 21 sec (control 13 sec); PTTK: 57 sec (control 35 sec).
(a) Give two investigations which would be diagnostically useful.
(b) What is the likely haematological diagnosis?

6. A 63-year-old man is investigated for breathlessness.
Vital capacity: 2.1l (3.9–5.0l); FEV₁ : 1.6l (2.3–3.6l); Total Lung Capacity (TLC): 4.6l (5.6–7.5l); Transfer factor (DLCO): 7.7 (26mlCO/min/Hg); Compliance: 0.13 l/cmH₂0 (>0.2 l/cm).
(a) What abnormality is demonstrated?
(b) Give three possible causes.

7. A 42-year-old man was admitted following onset of pleuritic chest pain.
Hb: 7.4g/dl (7.4g/100ml); PCV: 0.27 (27%); MCV: 72fl (72μm³); WBC: 12.4 × 10⁹/l (12,400/mm³); Neutrophils: 68%; Lymphocytes: 22%; Monocytes: 2%; Basophils: 6%; Platelets: 1,050 × 10⁹/l (1,050,000/mm³); Ferritin: 12μg/100ml.
(a) List two further helpful investigations at this stage.
(b) Suggest two possible diagnoses.

8. A 35-year-old woman complained of lassitude and polyuria.
Hb: 14.4g/dl (14.4g/100ml); ESR: 6mm/h; Urea: 3.6mmol/l (22mg/100ml); Ca: 3.01mmol/l (11.8mg/100ml); PO4: 1.87mmol/l (6.01mg/100ml); Albumin: 43g/l (4.3g/100ml); PTH: <0.1ng/ml; T4: 98nmol/l.
(a) List three investigations which would assist in establishing the diagnosis.
(b) Suggest two possible diagnoses.

9. A 15-year-old girl is investigated because of short stature. On examination, pubertal development is absent. A combined anterior pituitary function test is carried out (insulin: 0.15u/kg iv, TRH: 200μg iv, LHRH: 100μg iv).

Time (min)	Glucose mmol/l	Cortisol nmol/l	GH mU/l	TSH mU/l	LH U/l	FSH U/l
0	4.6	370	<1	1.5	>25	>50
15	2.1	410	18			
30	0.8	470	24	12.2	>25	>50
45	2.9	660	16			
60	3.8	588	8	6.8	>25	>50
90	4.1	475	4			

(a) Suggest a probable diagnosis.
(b) List one confirmatory investigation.

10. A 65-year-old man was investigated following a seizure.
Urea: 5.6mmol/l (35mg/100ml); Sodium: 112mmol/l (112mEq/l); Potassium: 3.9mmol/l (3.9mEq/l); Plasma osmolality: 238mOsm/kg; Urinary osmolality: 560mOsm/kg.
Suggest two possible underlying causes for the abnormality.

Answers

1. Rheumatoid arthritis ★★★★
   Psoriatic arthropathy 0
   Osteoarthritis 0
   There is a boutonnière deformity and nailfold vasculitic lesions.

2. (a) Oral candidiasis ★★★★
       Infectious mononucleosis 0
   (b) Diabetes mellitus ★★★★
       Cytotoxic chemotherapy ★★★★
       Immunosuppression ★★★★
       Antibiotic chemotherapy ★★★★

3. Branch retinal vein occlusion ★★★★
   Segmented retinal artery occlusion ★
   There has been retinal vascular leakage, haemorrhage and oedema in the affected area. Retinal venous occlusion is associated with diabetes mellitus, hypertension and hyperviscosity states. Most branch retinal vein occlusions occur in the temporal retina at arteriovenous crossings in patients with systemic hypertension or arteriosclerosis.

4. Dermatomyositis ★★★★
   Systemic lupus erythematosus ★
   Exfoliative dermatitis ★
   Eczema 0
   The rash can mimic exfoliative dermatitis. There is erythema over the dorsal and metacarpophalangeal joints, with a tendency for the rash to be streaked along the extensor tendons. This pattern is characteristic of dermatomyositis and is to be distinguished from that of lupus erythematosus where the knuckles are spared.

5. Neurofibromatosis ★★★★
   Dermocellular naevi 0
   Cutaneous manifestations of neurofibromatosis include multiple skin-coloured pedunculated tumours and subcutaneous nodules along nerve sheaths. Café-au-lait spots may be present at birth. Skin tumours become more numerous throughout life and can arise in all tissues, including bone and lung, in which they cause cystic lesions. Scoliosis, kyphoscoliosis with gibbus formation, lordosis and pseudoarthrosis may occur. Associations include bilateral acoustic neuromas, gliomas of the optic nerve, nodules in the iris, hamartomas of the retina and phaeochromocytoma.

6. Cutaneous amyloidosis ★★★★
   Morphoea ★
   The usual cutaneous lesions in amyloidosis consist of slightly raised waxy papules or plaques which usually cluster in the axillary folds, in the anal or inguinal region, the face and neck, as well as in mucosal areas such as the ear or tongue. Gentle rubbing of the overlying skin usually causes purpura.

7. Polycythaemia rubra vera (PRV) ★★★★
   Polycythaemia ★
   There is facial plethora and injection of the mucous membranes with a 'magenta' tongue. Splenomegaly is seen in 75% of PRV at presentation. The spleen is firm and non-tender, containing a large amount of extramedullary haemopoietic tissue where, in particular, excessive granulo- and thrombopoiesis occur.

8. Thalassaemia major ★★★★
   Severe osteoporosis 0
   The marrow has expanded at the expense of the cortex which becomes thin. There is severe osteopenia, with loss of tubulation of bones in the feet, and a coarsened trabecular pattern with reduced trabecular numbers. Spinal changes consist of generalised osteopenia and biconcavity of the vertebral bodies.

9. Necrobiosis lipoidica ★★★★

Eczema 0
Bowen's disease 0
Necrobiosis lipoidica occurs more frequently in females than in males, and may antedate other clinical signs and symptoms of diabetes. This lesion has ulcerated. When mature, the lesion is painless and consists of an area of atrophic skin, usually pigmented with small telangiectasia around the border. It may follow trauma.

10. B12 deficiency ★★★★
    Folic acid deficiency ★★★★
    A giant and abnormally shaped metamyelocyte is present. Other changes seen in megaloblastic anaemia include a hypercellular marrow with large erythroblasts which show failure of nuclear maturation, maintaining an open, fine, primitive chromatin pattern but normal haemoglobinisation. Peripheral blood film abnormalities would include oval macrocytosis, low reticulocyte count, reduced total white cells and platelets, and hypersegmented neutrophils (nuclei with six or more lobes).

11. Eruptive xanthomas ★★★★
    Gouty tophi 0
    This is associated with hypertriglyceridaemia. Eruptive xanthomata are found in type I, IIb, IV and V hyperlipidaemias. Diabetes mellitus should be sought. A sudden eruption of profuse xanthomas may occur in liver disease with jaundice, nephrotic syndrome, myxoedema and chronic pancreatitis.

12. Double contrast barium enema ★★★★
    Carcinoma of the caecum ★★★★
    A typical 'apple core' lesion is shown in this double contrast barium enema.

13. Asbestosis ★★★★
    Pleural fibromas 0
    Pulmonary metastases 0
    Both pleural and parenchymal abnormalities may occur in asbestosis. In the pleura, plaque formation (seen here), diffuse pleural thickening, calcification and effusions occur. Parenchymal abnormalities include lower zone reticulation, progressing to widespread interstitial fibrosis.

14. Cutaneous sarcoidosis ★★★★
    Cutaneous tubercle ★
    Skin involvement in sarcoidosis includes lupus pernio, maculo-papular eruptions, plaques, nodules and scar granulomas.

15. Paget's disease of the forearm ★★★★
    Quervain's disease (tenovaginitis of radial styloid) ★
    There is bowing of the radius.

16. Phlyctenular conjunctivis ★★★★
    Iritis ★
    This is secondary to Crohn's disease. Ocular manifestations in this condition include an intense conjunctivitis and uveitis/iritis. Phlyctenular keratoconjunctivitis can also occur as a rare allergic external ocular inflammation observed in children at the time of primary tuberculous infection, and characterised by small blisters (phlyctenules) at the junction of the conjunctiva and cornea.

17. Primary biliary sclerosis ★★★★
    Alcoholic hepatitis 0
    The first stage of the disease is characterized by inflammatory destruction of intrahepatic bile ducts by lymphocytes, monocyte macrophages and plasma cells.

18. Medullary sponge kidney ★★★★
    Polycystic kidneys 0
    This is a disorder of the intrapyramidal or intrapapillary segments of the renal collecting tubules, characterised by ectasia of collecting tubules sometimes to the point of actual cyst formation.

Complications include stone formation, infection and renal tubular acidosis. Hypercalciuria occurs in 40% of cases.

19. *Plasmodium vivax* infection ★★★★
    Malaria ★★
    In *P. vivax*, which causes benign tertian malaria, the ring forms are large and stout, often measuring one third of the red cell. The infected erythrocytes are larger than normal, and Schüffner's dots can be identified. The mature schizont contains 12-24 chromatin dots, and the parasite cytoplasm almost fills the red blood cells. The female gametocyte is globular in shape.

20. Secondary syphilis ★★★★
    Pityriasis rosea ★
    Toxic erythema ★
    Psoriasis 0
    There are smooth-topped or scaly, symmetrical brownish papules on the soles of the foot. Patchy loss of scalp hair may also be present. Syphilis serology is strongly positive in secondary syphilis.

ANSWERS TO CASE STUDIES

Case I

1. Reticulocyte count ★★★★
   Bone marrow aspirate for microscopy and culture ★★★★
   Thick blood film for malarial parasites ★★★★
   Echocardiogram ★★★★
   Blood cultures ★★★★
   Brucella titres ★★
   CT scan of abdomen ★★
   Viral antibody screen, e.g. CMV, EBV ★★
   Immunoglobulin electrophoresis ★★
   Iron and total iron binding capacity ★★
   Faecal occult blood ★★
   Upper/lower GI endoscopy ★★

2. Visceral leishmaniasis ★★★★
   Lymphoma, e.g. Hodgkin's disease ★★★
   Tuberculosis ★★
   Subacute bacterial endocarditis ★★
   Malaria ★
   This patient was suffering from visceral leishmaniasis. This diagnosis must be suspected in any patient living in, or having visited an endemic area, who has a prolonged fever. The diagnosis is likely with the following physical signs: Splenomegaly, granulocytopenia, anaemia and hyper-globulinaemia. The diagnosis is best made by needle aspiration of bone marrow, spleen, liver or lymph nodes, to look for the parasite. Antileishmanial antibodies can be demonstrated by indirect immunofluorescence of promastigotes in over 90% of cases. The leishmanin test is negative in cases of visceral leishmaniasis, but becomes positive after recovery. Diseases which can be confused with visceral leishmaniasis include:
   Aleukaemic leukaemia;
   Tropical splenomegaly syndrome (IgM↑↑);
   Cirrhosis with portal hypertension and hypersplenism;
   Miliary tuberculosis;
   Schistosomiasis;
   Brucellosis;
   Malaria;
   Bacterial endocarditis.

Case II

1. Myocardial biopsy ★★★★
   24h ECG to document rhythm disorders ★★★★
   ASO titre ★★★★
   Echocardiogram ★★★★
   Nuclear cardiac angiogram ★★★★
   Viral antibodies ★★ Blood cultures ★★

   Thyroxine measurement ★★
   Triiodothyronine measurement ★★

2. Congestive cardiomyopathy ★★★★
   Viral myocarditis ★★★★
   Rheumatic heart disease (acute with myocarditis) ★★★★
   Glue-sniffers' heart (cardiomyopathy) ★★★★
   Congestive cardiomyopathy may be considered as a syndrome of isolated cardiomegaly with dilated ventricles, inappropriate hypertrophy and heart failure. The cause is unknown, but a number of predisposing factors have been speculated upon: systemic hypertension, pregnancy and the puerperium, immunological disorders, viral infections, alcohol, and certain drugs such as daunorubicin, toxic agents such as cobalt, and solvent abuse. Chagas' disease, caused by *Trypanosoma cruzei*, may cause an acute congestive cardiomyopathy, and the infective organism can be readily demonstrated in the myocardium. In making the diagnosis, rare specific heart muscle disease must be excluded, such as systemic sclerosis, SLE, polyarteritis, haemochromatosis, generalised myopathy, Friedreich's ataxia and sarcoidosis.

Case III

1. X-ray of the dorsal vertebrae ★★★★
   Myelography ★★★★
   Examination of CSF for cells, protein, oligoclonal bands ★★★★
   Bone scan ★★★★
   VDRL TPHA ★★
   Magnetic Resonance Imaging (MRI) of dorsal spinal cord ★★
   Visual evoked responses ★★

2. Extrinsic cord compression of the level of D6-7.
      The lesion is behaving like a Brown-Séquard
      syndrome ★★★★
   Multiple sclerosis ★★
   Transverse myelitis ★★

Case IV

1. Biopsy and culture of orbital swelling ★★★★
   Muscle biopsy/temporal artery biopsy ★★★★
   Biopsy of skin lesion ★★★★
   HBsAg ★★
   Visceral angiogram ★★
   CT scan of orbit ★★
   Barium meal, barium enema, CT scan of abdomen,
      to look for malignancy ★
   Thyroid autoantibodies 0

2. Polyarteritis nodosa ★★★★
   Wegener's granulomatosis ★★★★
   Vasculitis ★★★★
   The clinical features in this case suggest a vasculitic aetiology. Both polyarteritis nodosa and Wegener's granulomatosis could present with features of an 'orbital pseudotumour'. Wegener's granulomatosis is a necrotising granulomatous vasculitis which may exist in a generalised or limited form. Eye manifestations are common and occur in 40-50% of cases. Ocular involvement includes conjunctivitis, episcleritis, scleritis, corneoscleral ulceration, uveitis, optic neuritis, retinal artery occlusion and orbital involvement with proptosis from pseudotumour of the orbit, or orbital cellulitis.

Case V

1. Echocardiogram ★★★★
   Blood cultures ★★★★
   CT scan of the head to exclude cerebral abscess ★★★★
   Radioisotope brain scan ★★
   Skull x-ray ★★

2. Cerebral abscess ★★★★
   Pyogenic septicaemia ★★
   Cortical vein thrombosis ★★

Answers

Since venous blood bypasses the normal filtering action of the lungs, emboli arising from the systemic veins may pass directly to the cerebral circulation. Patients with polycythaemia will have had previous occlusive microcirculatory episodes to the CNS. These predisposing factors are responsible for the 2–4% incidence of brain abscess in patients with cyanotic heart disease.

ANSWERS TO DATA INTERPRETATIONS

1. Acute anterolateral myocardial infarction ★★★★
   Ventricular premature beat ★★★★
   Sino - atrial arrest ★★★★

2. Presbyacusis ★★★★
   Sensory-neural deafness ★★
   There is a sloping sensory-neural hearing loss, typical of presbyacusis.

3. Right bundle branch block ★★★★
   Left axis deviation ★★★★
   Mobitz type II block ★★★★
   Trifascicular block ★★★★
   Left anterior hemiblock ★★★★
   Prolonged PR interval ★★★★

4. Cyanotic heart disease ★★★★
   Extensive bronchiectasis ★★
   Cystic fibrosis ★★★★
   In order of frequency, the commonest causes of cyanotic heart disease with R→L shunt are: Tetralogy of Fallot, complete or D-transposition of the great vessels, tricuspid atresia, and aortic and mitral atresia. Pulmonary A-V aneurysm/fistulae is a rare cause of cyanosis, and associated with Osler-Rendu-Weber syndrome.

5. (a) Examination of blood film for red cell fragmentation or schistocytes ★★★★
      Fibrinogen level (decreased) ★★★★
      Fibrin degradation products (FDP) ↑ ★★★★
      Factors V & VIII low ★
   (b) Disseminated intravascular coagulation ★★★★
      Arterial embolus 0
   Release of thromboplastic substances into the circulation and activation of the extrinsic clotting system can occur following extensive myocardial infarction. Other causes of DIC include: (a) Trauma – surgery, obstetric accidents; (b) Malignant disease – metastatic carcinomas, promyelocytic leukaemia; (c) Severe infection, e.g. Gram-negative septicaemia; (d) Burns; (e) Antigen-antibody reactions, e.g. severe immune haemolysis.

6. (a) Restrictive ventilatory defect ★★★★
      Mixed obstructive/restrictive defect 0
   (b) Sarcoidosis ★★★★
      Fibrosing alveolitis ★★★★
      Lymphangitis carcinomatosa ★★
      Severe pulmonary oedema ★★
   A restrictive pattern of respiratory function consists of a relatively normal FEV_1/FVC ratio, a relatively normal ratio of RV/TLC, but often a reduced PEF combined with a low TLC. There is usually associated low lung compliance ('stiff lungs'), and a low transfer factor for carbon monoxide.

7. (a) Chest X-ray ★★★★
      Ventilation-perfusion lung scan ★★★★
      Bone marrow examination ★★★★
      Gastroscopy/colonoscopy ★★★★
      Upper and lower GI tract barium studies ★★★★
      Reticulocyte count ★★★★
      Electrocardiogram ★★
      Faecal occult bloods ★★

   (b) Iron deficiency anaemia from chronic bleeding ★★★★
      Essential thrombocythaemia ★★★★
   Causes of secondary thrombocytosis include: (a) Reactive – to blood loss, haemolysis; (b) Post-splenectomy; (c) In association with malignancy and chronic inflammatory disease states, e.g. rheumatoid arthritis. Essential thrombocythaemia is a myeloproliferative disorder with increased platelet production (>1000 × 10⁹/l). Platelet aggregation *in vitro* is often impaired. The blood film shows large and/or atypical platelets, and sometimes megakaryocyte fragments. The bone marrow shows increased megakaryocyte numbers. Splenomegaly is usual, as are pathological haemorrhages and thromboembolic episodes.

8. (a) Chest X-ray ★★★★
      Bone scan ★★★★
      Vitamin D level ★★★★
      Hydrocortisone suppression test ★★★★
      ACE level ★★
      Liver biopsy ★★
      Kveim test ★★
      Mantoux test ★★
      24 hour urinary calcium ★★
      Thyroid function tests ★★
   (b) Vitamin D intoxication ★★★★
      Sarcoidosis ★★★★
      Malignancy ★★★★
      Milk alkali syndrome ★★★★
      Thyrotoxicosis ★★★★
   Hypercalcaemia may occur in granulomatous disorders such as sarcoidosis, beryllium and zirconium toxicity, because of the capacity of granulomatous tissue to synthesise 1,25 dihydroxy-cholecalciferol. Neoplasms associated with hypercalcaemia include myeloma, and breast, lung, cervical and renal carcinomas.

9. (a) Turner's syndrome (46XO) ★★★★
      Pure gonadal dysgenesis ★★★★
      Primary ovarian failure ★★
      Resistant ovary syndrome ★★
   (b) Karyotype ★★★★
      Buccal smear ★★
      Laparoscopy and ovarian biopsy ★★
      Ovarian autoantibodies ★★
      Serum oestradiol ★★
   Primary amenorrhoea, together with short stature, should always suggest the possibility of Turner's syndrome (gonadal dysgenesis). This may be associated with an XO chromosomal abnormality, an XX/XO or some other (XO/XXX; XO/XX/XXX) mosaicism, or structural anomalies of the X chromosome (e.g. 46-isochromosome Xp-, Xq-). Turner's syndrome has a frequency of 1:5000 live births. In general, aplasia or hypoplasia of the ovaries (ovarian streaks) is present.

10. Ca bronchus with ADH production ★★★★
    Head injury ★★★★
    Hypothyroidism ★★★★
    Pulmonary tuberculosis ★★
    Other causes of inappropriate ADH secretion include: cerebrovascular disease, encephalitis, poliomyelitis, the Guillain-Barré syndrome, and acute intermittent porphyria. The simplest treatment is water restriction to 500ml daily. With coma and convulsions, 500ml of hypertonic (3%) saline will rapidly, but temporarily, improve the situation.

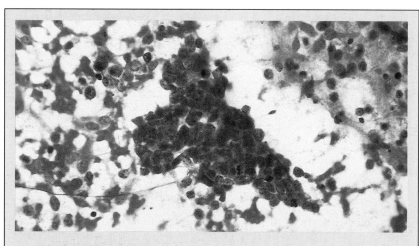

1. These cells were found in the sputum of a 54-year-old man with rapid weight loss. What is the diagnosis?

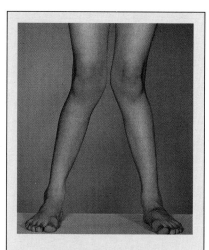

2. List three investigations which would be useful in determining the cause of this appearance.

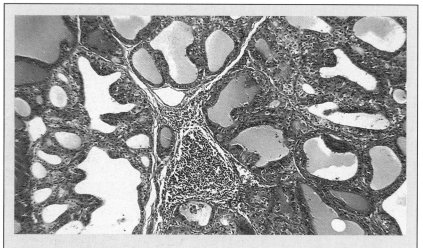

3. What is the diagnosis?

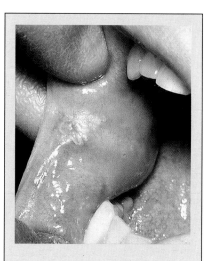

4. What is the diagnosis?

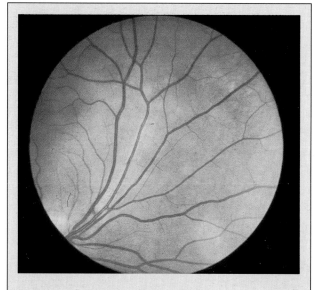

5. This lesion was an incidental finding. What is the diagnosis?

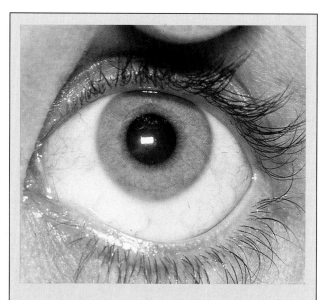

6. This is the eye of a 43-year-old woman with a long history of pathological bone fractures. What is the most likely underlying diagnosis?

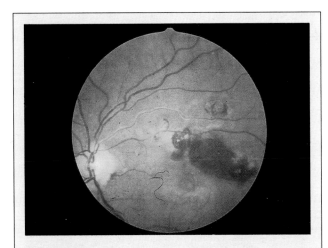

7. This the fundus of a 12-year-old black child who presented with a six month history of non-progressive visual loss. What is the diagnosis?

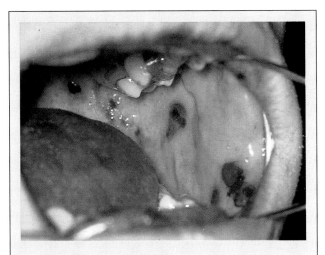

8. What is the most likely cause of this appearance?

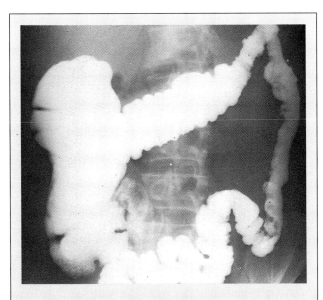

9. This barium enema was performed in a 75-year-old man three days after an acute bout of abdominal pain. What is the diagnosis?

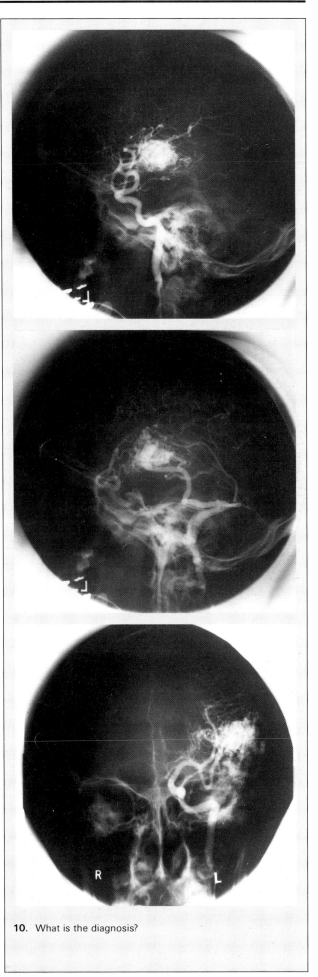

10. What is the diagnosis?

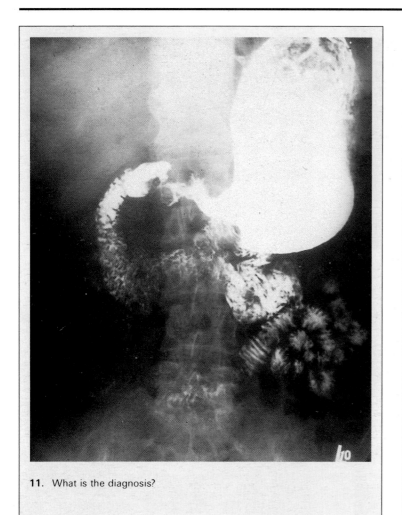

11. What is the diagnosis?

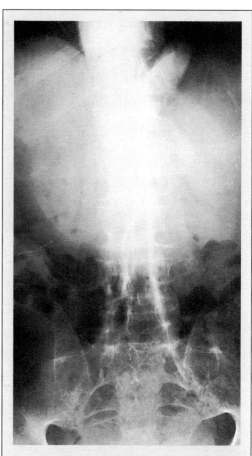

12. List two abnormalities on this radiograph. What is the diagnosis?

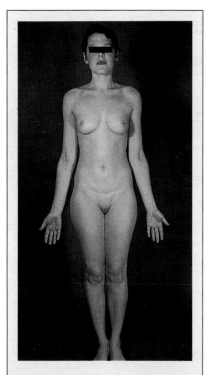

13. This woman presented with primary amenorrhoea. What is the diagnosis?

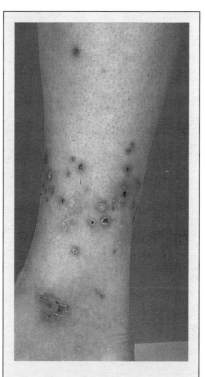

14. These lesions had been present on the legs of this diabetic patient for two months. What is the diagnosis?

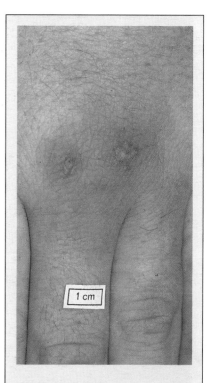

15. These lesions were found in the knuckles of a 35-year-old man with a monoarticular arthritis. What is the likely diagnosis?

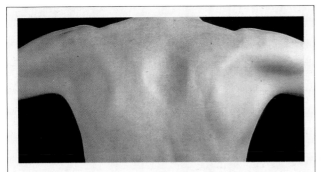

16. List three possible causes for this appearance.

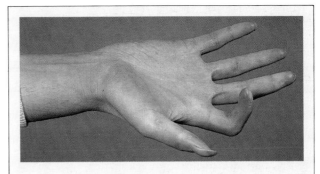

17. What is the diagnosis?

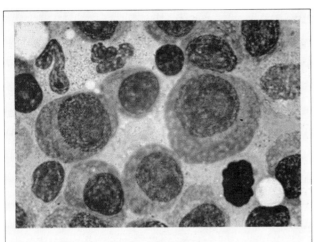

18. This is the appearance of a bone marrow aspirate from a patient with ESR of 110mm/h.
What is the diagnosis?

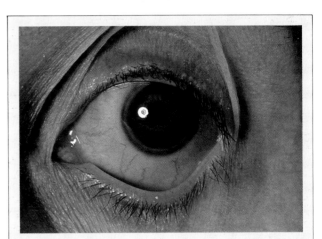

19. List two physical signs and two possible underlying diagnoses.

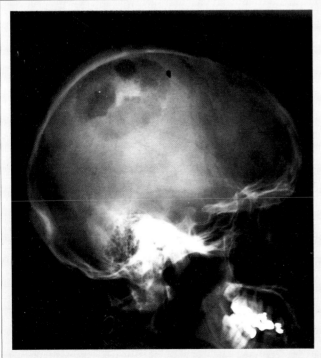
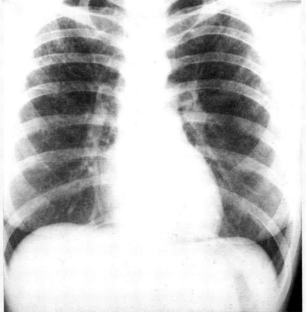

20. These are the skull and chest radiographs of a 30-year-old woman who was under investigation for pain in the hip.
   (a) What abnormality is seen in (I) the skull and (II) the chest?
   (b) Suggest a likely diagnosis.

CASE I

An urgent medical opinion was requested for a 16-year-old girl who had recently undergone an appendicectomy operation. She had apparently been well until four months prior to admission, when she began to experience frequent loose bowel motions, not associated with abdominal pain. Two days before admission, she had developed localised pain in the right iliac fossa, associated with some vomiting and fever. A diagnosis of appendicitis was made, and the patient was referred to hospital for a surgical opinion. The surgical team proceeded to a routine appendicectomy. The excised appendix showed evidence of active inflammation. The patient was well immediately after the operation, but within 24 hours became delirious, with an unexplained temperature of 39°C. She became dehydrated, with persistent tachycardia.

On examination, the patient looked unwell and dehydrated. Pulse 140/min, blood pressure 140/60mmHg. Her mucous membranes were dry, and the eyeballs appeared sunken. Tissue turgor was diminished. A smooth goitre was noted. Her chest was clear, but examination of the heart revealed an ejection systolic murmur, best heard at the base of the heart, and a third sound best heard at the apex. Apart from her tender abdominal incision, there were no other physical signs elicited in the abdomen. Bowel sounds were present. Examination of the nervous system revealed some evidence of muscle wasting. The reflexes were brisk, and the plantar responses were bilaterally flexor.

Investigations

HAEMATOLOGY
Hb: 15.6g/dl (15.6g/100ml); MCV: 78fl (78μm³); WBC: 6.8 × 10⁹/l (6,800/mm); Neutrophils: 80%; ESR: 16mm/h.

BIOCHEMISTRY & RADIOLOGY
Urea: 17.4mmol/l (105mg/100); Creatinine: 0.13mmol/l (1.5mg/100ml); Sodium: 145mmol/l (145mEq/l); Potassium: 4.8mmol/l (4.8mEq/l); Bicarbonate: 28mmol/l (28mEq/l); Chloride: 108mmol/l (108mEq/l); Bilirubin: 14μmol/l (0.82mg/100ml); Alkaline phosphatase: 235iu/l (30.5KAU/100ml); Total protein: 83g/l (8.3g/100ml); Calcium: 2.98mmol/l (11.7mg/100ml); Phosphate: 1.26mmol/l (4.04mg/100ml); Serum glutamic oxaloacetic transaminase (SGOT) 33iu/l; Urinanalysis: some granular casts seen, but otherwise normal; CXR: normal heart size, lungs clear; ECG: sinus tachycardia, normal axis, no QRS or ST segment abnormalities.

1. List three investigations which would assist in the patients's management.

2. What is the most likely diagnosis?

CASE II

A 48-year-old plumber was admitted to hospital after being found in a delirious state at home. He was a single man, and had a long history of alcohol abuse, often totalling ten pints a day. A neighbour, who accompanied him to hospital, gave a history that over the previous fortnight the patient had 'gone off his food', and during the week prior to admission had had profuse yellow diarrhoea which, over the last two days, was associated with vomiting. He had lost over 7kg in weight. In his past, he had been in reasonably good health and had never suffered any serious illnesses.

On examination, he was an ill-looking man with a pyrexia of 37.8°C. He was clinically dehydrated, and disorientated in time and place. There was an alcoholic smell in his breath. Two spider naevi were noted over his upper trunk, and his palms were erythematous. There was no jaundice or liver flap. Examination of the heart and lungs was unremarkable, except for a tachycardia of 110/min. Blood pressure was 120/75mmHg. There was clinical evidence of a right pleural effusion. Abdominal examination revealed tender hepatomegaly, with the liver edge 5cm palpable below the right costal margin. The epigastrium was particularly tender to palpation. The central nervous system examination, apart from the delirious state, was unremarkable. The fundi were normal, and plantar reflexes were bilaterally flexor.

Investigations

HAEMATOLOGY
Hb: 12.8g/dl (12.8g/100ml); MCV: 103fl (103μm³); WBC: 15.6 × 10⁹/l (15,600/mm³); Neutrophils: 84%; ESR: 84mm/h.

BIOCHEMISTRY & RADIOLOGY
Urea: 4.8mmol/l (25mg/100ml); Creatinine: 0.08mmol/l (0.9mg/100ml); Sodium: 130mmol/l (130mEq/l); Potassium: 2.9mmol/l (2.9mEq/l); Chloride: 93mmol/l (89mEq/l); Bicarbonate: 26mmol/l (22mEq/l); Bilirubin: 24μmol/l (1.41mg/100ml); Alkaline phosphatase: 272iu/l (36KAU/100ml); SGOT: 64iu/l; Serum glutamic pyruvic transaminase (SGPT): 78iu/l; Total protein: 54g/l (5.4g/100ml); Albumin: 26g/l (2.6g/100ml); Calcium: 2.01mmol/l (7.9mg/100ml); Phosphate: 0.94mmol/l (3.02mg/100ml); CXR: There is a moderate right-sided pleural effusion.

1. List three diagnostically useful investigations.

2. What is the most likely diagnosis?

CASE III

A 73-year-old patient complained of a painless onset of her tongue feeling 'thick and peculiar'. Recently, after eating, she had found it almost impossible to talk. There was no hoarseness or dysphagia, but she had become conscious of the act of swallowing, and complained that while chewing her food particles tended to lodge between her cheeks and gums. When drinking she had to press the cup against her tongue, otherwise the contents would be spilt. There was no nasal regurgitation of fluid. In her medical history, she had been suffering from rheumatoid arthritis since the age of 52, which had been treated with steroids and recently with penicillamine. She also suffered from mild hypertension, managed with propranolol. The present symptoms had been gradually developing over six weeks. Systemic enquiry was otherwise unremarkable.

On examination, the only abnormal physical sign elicited was that she could not completely close her left eye. Pulse was 64/min regular, blood pressure 160/90mmHg. The chest was clear, and heart sounds were normal except for an accentuated aortic second sound. There was no lymphadenopathy; abdominal and pelvic examinations were unremarkable. In the central nervous system, cranial nerves were intact except for the inability to close her left eye fully. Tone, power, coordination reflexes were all preserved, and plantars were bilaterally flexor.

1. List three diagnostically useful investigations.

2. What is the most likely diagnosis?

CASE IV

A 38-year-old man was admitted as an emergency for investigation of dyspnoea. One week previously, he was sailing in a boat when he decided to dive in the river for a swim. Upon surfacing, he felt intensely dyspnoeic and was therefore scarcely able to reach the river bank. He was usually very fit, and had been a jogger for many years. On the following day, he once again attempted to swim, but found that he became breathless as soon as the water line reached just above his hip level; at this point he became much more dyspnoeic and had to return to the shore. There, his breathlessness disappeared and he felt quite normal. Recently, he had experienced mild orthopnoea at night. In his past medical history, the man had been fit, with no indication of lung disease.

On examination, the patient looked fit, with no evidence of clubbing or anaemia. Pulse 80/min regular, blood pressure 120/80mmHG. The jugulovenous pulse was normal. Examination of the head and neck was unremarkable, and it was noted that the patient was not using his accessory muscles for respiration. The trachea was central, and examination of the chest was entirely normal. Cardiovascular, abdominal and central nervous system examinations were all normal, except for mild bilateral winging of the scapulae. There was no sensory abnormality.

Investigations

HAEMATOLOGY
Hb: 14.6g/dl (14.6g/100ml); MCV: 90fl (90μm^3); MCH: 27pg (27$\mu\mu$g); WBC: 6.4 × 10^9/l (6,400/mm^3); ESR: 12mm/h.

BIOCHEMISTRY
Urea: 4.6mmol/l (24mg/100ml); Creatinine: 0.09mmol/l; Sodium: 138mmol/l (138mEq/l); Potassium: 3.9mmol/l (3.9 mEq/l); Bicarbonate: 26mmol/l (26mEq/l); Chloride: 98mmol/l (98mEq/l); Liver function tests: normal; CPK: 32iu/l; Urinanalysis: no abnormalities seen.

RADIOLOGY & SPECIAL INVESTIGATIONS
CXR: no pulmonary or cardiac abnormalities seen; ECG: sinus rhythm, normal QRS complexes, no T-wave abnormalities; Lung function tests: vital capacity; 4.1 standing (predicted 3.9–5.2); 2.61 lying (predicted 3.5–4.8); FEV$_1$/FVC ratio: 75% (predicted 75–90%).

1. Suggest three investigations which would assist in establishing a diagnosis.

2. What is the most likely diagnosis?

CASE V

A 27-year-old woman had been perfectly well until two weeks prior to admission, when she developed peripheral oedema and progressive exertional dyspnoea. She began to experience diffuse headaches, and noticed that her urine had become cloudy and occasionally dark. Her past medical history was unremarkable, except that she had suffered from congenital deafness.

On examination, her temperature was 37.8°C, her pulse 80/min, and blood pressure 180/130mmHg. There was clear peripheral oedema, involving the legs and the sacral region. Her jugulovenous pulse was raised 10cm, and examination of the lungs revealed dullness in both bases, with crackles present on inspiration. The heart was clinically enlarged, and auscultation of the left sternal border revealed an ejection systolic murmur with fixed splitting of the second sound. Her thumbs were noted to be congenitally short in both hands.

Investigations

HAEMATOLOGY
Hb: 11.4g/dl (11.4g/100ml); PCV: 0.32 (32%); WBC: 11 × 10^9/l (11,000/mm^3); Neutrophils: 82%; Lymphocytes: 7%; Platelets: 250 × 10^9/l (250,000/mm^3); ESR: 60mm/h.

BIOCHEMISTRY & RADIOLOGY
Prothrombin time: 11sec (control 12sec); Urea: 16.4mmol/l (100mg/100ml); Creatinine: 211μmol/l (2.38mg/100ml); Sodium: 132mmol/l (132mEq/l); Potassium: 4mmol/l (4mEq/l); Bicarbonate: 14mmol/l (14mEq/l); Calcium: 2.1μmol (8.23mg/100ml); Phosphate: 1.6mmol/l (5.79mg/100ml); Bilirubin: 17μmol/l (1mg/100ml); Uric acid: 0.5mmol/l (8.3mg/100ml); SGOT: 22iu/l; Alkaline phosphatase: 104iu/l (14KAU/100ml); Urinanalysis: protein +++, red cells +, 5 granular casts high powered field; CXR: Cardiomegaly, bilateral pleural effusions, interstitial pulmonary oedema.

1. List five steps which are required in her management at presentation.

2. List three diagnoses.

Data Interpretations

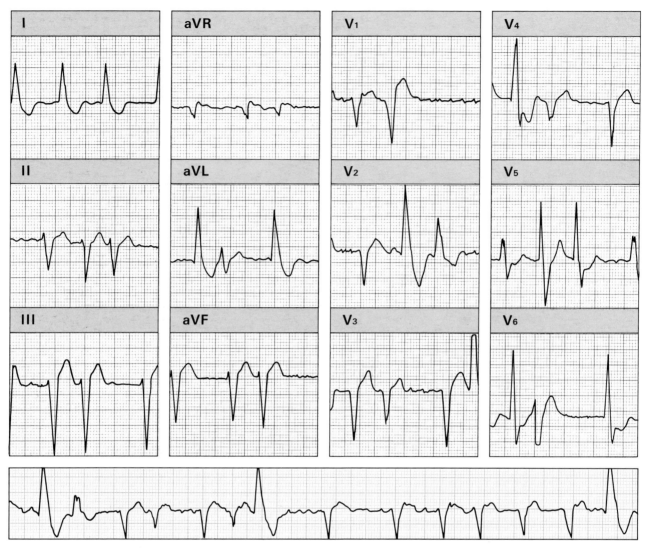

1. What abnormalities are present on this electrocardiogram?

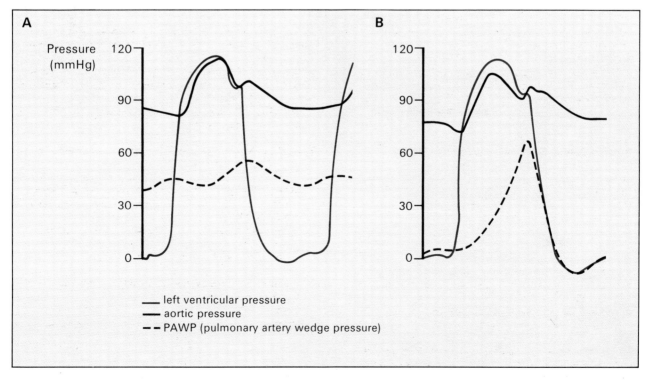

left ventricular pressure
aortic pressure
PAWP (pulmonary artery wedge pressure)

2. What diagnoses would account for the cardiac catheter pressure tracings shown in **A** and **B**?

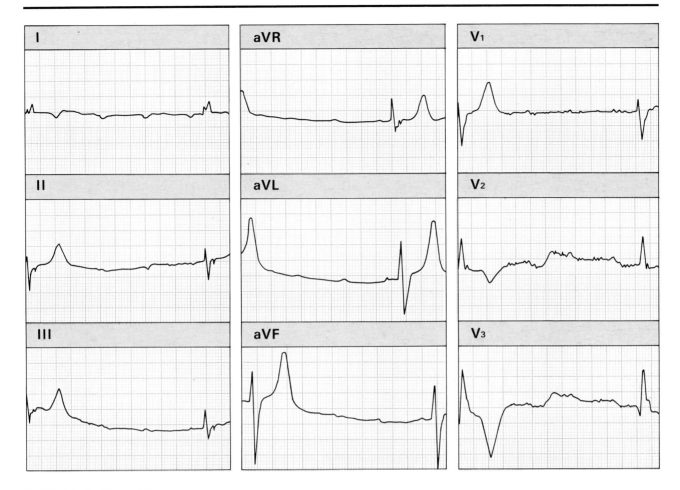

3. What is the diagnosis?

4. An 85-year-old lady, under treatment for a chest infection, developed an acute and exquisitely tender swelling of the wrist joint. This was aspirated.
   Fluid turbid; Neutrophils: +++; Weakly positive, birefringent crystals noted within neutrophils; Peripheral WBC: 14×10^9/l (14,000/mm³); Neutrophils: 75%.
   (a) What is the most probable diagnosis?
   (b) Suggest one investigation which would help in obtaining a diagnosis.

5. A 62-year-old woman presented with an eight-week history of tiredness and increasing dyspnoea. The cardiac catheter data were as follows:

	PRESSURES (mmHg)	
	Phasic	Mean
Right atrium	—	5
Right ventricle	33/8	—
Pulmonary artery	33/20	25
Pul Cap Wedge	—	18
Left ventricle	214/6	—
LVEDP	22	—
Aorta	155/80	
Cardiac output	3.9 l/min	

   What is the diagnosis?

6. A 24-year-old woman complained of flitting arthralgia.
   Hb: 12.4g/dl (12.4g/100ml); ESR: 32mm/h; RA latex test: negative; VDRL: positive.
   (a) List two useful diagnostic investigations.
   (b) Suggest two possible diagnoses.

7. A 23-year-old labourer required 18 units of blood following stab wounds in the abdomen and chest. Five weeks later he had the following blood count:
   Hb: 11.4g/dl (11.4g/100ml); PCV: 0.37 (37%); MCV: 84fl

(84μm³); Platelets: 68×10^9/l (68,000/mm³); WBC: 11.2×10^9/l (11,200/mm³); Polychromasia: ++; Reactive lymphocytes: 27%.
   (a) Suggest three further investigations which would clarify the underlying diagnosis.
   (b) Suggest one possible explanation for the above findings.

8. At a follow-up visit to Outpatients, an 18-year-old woman on treatment for intestinal Crohn's disease has the following blood count:
   Hb: 9.3g/dl (9.3g/100ml); Reticulocytes: 4.8%; Blood film: Red cell fragmentation; Heinz bodies: ++ after incubation of blood for 36 hours.
   (a) What is the haematological diagnosis?
   (b) Suggest a likely cause.

9. A 36-year-old woman complains of severe difficulty with rising from her chair.
   Urea: 6.7mmol/l (35mg/100ml); Calcium: 1.76mmol/l (6.9mg/100ml); PO₄: 0.96mmol/l (3.1mg/100ml); Alkaline phosphatase: 155iu/l; Albumin: 31g/l (3.1g/100ml); Red cell folate: 68μg/l.
   (a) List two investigations which would be diagnostically useful.
   (b) Suggest a likely cause for these findings.

10. Give three possible causes for the following glucose tolerance test (75g orally).

Time (min)	Glucose (mmol/l)	GH (mU/l)
0	4.5	8
30	9.6	14.6
60	11.5	18.4
90	8.4	12.2
120	6.8	6.4

Answers

1. Oat cell carcinoma ★★★★
Small cell carcinoma ★★★★
Pneumocystis carinii 0
The cancerous cells are highly cellular and the individual cells typically round. Most of the cell is occupied by nucleus.

2. Wrist X-ray ★★★★
Urinary calcium estimation (low) ★★★★
Serum alkaline phosphatase ★★★★
Plasma 1,25 dihydroxy-cholecalciferol ★★★★
Plasma phosphate ★★★★
These are the 'knock-knee' appearances of rickets. The wrist X-ray characteristically shows an ill-defined epiphysis with a widened growth plate, with widening, fraying and cupping of the metaphysis.

3. Graves' disease ★★★★
Hashimoto's thyroiditis 0
This is the typical histological picture in Graves' disease. The epithelium is tall, columnar and follicular, and may be unfolded. There is scalloping of the colloid, associated with varying degrees of lymphocytic infiltration.

4. Secondary syphilis ★★★★
Leucoplakia ★
Trauma ★
Lichen planus 0
These snail-track ulcers are superficial erosions covered by a thin, white slough, which is easily scraped off. They are usually painless, and treponemes abound in these lesions.

5. Choroidal naevus ★★★★
Melanoma 0
Choroidal naevi are common and occur in about 10% of the caucasian population, most commonly in the posterior pole. They have a low malignant potential, the change to malignancy being about 1 in 5000 per year. They typically are a slate-grey colour, with well-defined borders. About 5% are amelanotic. Multiple or bilateral naevi are often seen in neurofibromatosis. A diameter of 10mm, or more than minimal elevation of the overlying retina, suggests malignant change within a naevus.

6. Gaucher's disease ★★★★
Pingueculae ★
Pingueculae are raised yellowish patches which gradually enlarge until they abut the cornea, but do not encroach on it. Histologically, they are formed by elastic degeneration of collagen within the substantia propria. Pingueculae are characteristic of Gaucher's disease. The disease is caused by abnormal accumulation of glucocerebrosides in reticuloendothelial cells, secondary to glucosyl-ceramide-β-glucosidase deficiency. The increasing mass of storage cells accounts for most of the clinical manifestations of the disease, including hepato-splenomegaly, lymph node enlargement and bone lesions.

7. Toxocariasis ★★★★
Toxoplasmosis ★★
Congenital syphilis ★★
Choroidoretinitis ★★
Toxocara (nematode) has its reservoir especially in young puppies, and the ova persist for long periods in contaminated soil. A pulmonary infiltrate, transient eosinophilia, fever and tender hepatomegaly may be present in the acute stages of the disease. The granulomatous endophthalmitis may be observed in older children and adults, and is typically unilateral and occurs in the absence of other clinical manifestations of toxocariasis. Decreased visual acuity or strabismus brings the patient to the physician.

8. Severe thrombocytopenia ★★★★
Disseminated intravascular coagulation ★★
Severe thrombocytopenia is characterised by spontaneous skin purpura, mucosal haemorrhage and prolonged bleeding after trauma, and menorrhagia in women. Causes are classified by:
(a) Failure of platelet production (e.g. drugs, infections); part of general marrow failure (e.g. aplastic anaemia, leukaemia, marrow infiltration). (b) Increased platelet destruction: ITP, drug-induced, DIC. (c) Abnormal destruction of platelets (e.g. splenomegaly).

9. Ischaemic colitis ★★★★
Ulcerative colitis ★
Lymphoma of colon 0
The wall of the descending colon is oedematous, the lumen narrow, with 'thumb printing'. This sign is not specific to ischaemic colitis, and is seen on barium enema with ulcerative colitis, Crohn's colitis, pseudomembranous colitis, amoebic colitis, schitosomiasis, lymphoma and colonic metastases.

10. Arteriovenous fistula/malformation ★★★★
Cerebral tumour 0
Such fistulae are usually congenital, and present in adult life. Plain radiography may show flecks of calcification with one or more characteristic ring shadows. They increase in size with age, and this proceeds more rapidly once adult blood pressure has been established. The communications between arteries and veins lie over the surface of the brain, but with increasing size extend into the brain substance in the manner of an inverted cone.

11. Chronic duodenal ulceration with scarring ★★★★
Gastric ulcer 0
Malabsorption 0

12. (a) Sacroiliitis ★★★★
Paraspinous ligament calcification ★★★★
(b) Ankylosing spondylitis ★★★★
Forestier's disease 0
Early changes in the sacroiliac joints include periarticular erosions, juxta-articular osteoporosis and absorption of subarticular bone. Serrated margins are present, and the joint shape is widened due to bone destruction; it soon becomes narrowed as a result of cartilage destruction. Eventually, there is complete ankylosis. Spinal changes include squaring of vertebrae, ligamentous ossification (of paraspinal ligaments), eventually leading to 'bamboo spine'. Atlantoaxial subluxation occurs in 2% of cases.

13. Testicular feminization ★★★★
Complete androgen resistance ★★★★
These are the classical appearances of testicular feminization.

14. Diabetic dermopathy ★★★★
Dermatitis artefacta ★
Furunculosis 0
The lesion has also been called 'spotted leg' or pigmented pretibial patches. They are usually precipitated by trauma; histologically, there is basilar hypermelanosis and slight proliferation of small blood vessels. Neuropathy, retinopathy and nephropathy are frequently associated.

15. Gonococcal septicaemia ★★★★
Staphylococcal septicaemia ★★
Vasculitis 0
Gonococcal bacteraemia is rare, and occurs predominantly in women. The features of disseminated gonococcal infection include variable fever, joint pains and a pustular eruption. Gonococci can usually be readily isolated from the genital tract, but with a lot more difficulty from blood cultures, joint fluid or the pustular rash.

16. Metabolic myopathy ★★★★
Limb girdle dystrophy ★★★★

Motor neurone disease ★★★★
Polymyositis ★★★★
Striking proximal myopathy may be seen with severe thyrotoxicosis and Cushing's syndrome. Limb girdle dystrophy is rare, with an incidence of 7:100,000 live births, and presentation in the third decade.

17. Scleroderma ★★★★
Systemic sclerosis ★★★★
This is sclerodactyly, telangiectasia, a flexion deformity of the forefinger, and pulp resorption. Calcinosis would be seen on X-ray, and chronic painful ulcers may develop.

18. Myeloma ★★★★
Chronic infection ★★★★
Chronic liver disease ★★
Collagen disease ★★
It is difficult to distinguish the plasma cell infiltrate of multiple myeloma from that of reactive plasmacytosis found in the above conditions.

19. (a) Blue sclerae ★★★★
    Arcus senilis ★★★★
    (b) Osteogenesis imperfecta ★★★★
    Iron deficiency anaemia ★★★★
    Hyperlipidaemia ★★★★

20. (a) Multiple punched out lytic lesions in the skull vault ★★★★
    Bilateral honey-combing in the upper and mid zones of the lung fields ★★★★
    (b) Histiocytosis X ★★★★
    Sarcoidosis ★
    Cystic fibrosis 0
    Patients with this disease usually present in childhood with the exception of eosinophilic granuloma, the most common and most benign form of this disease spectrum, which may present in later life. Bone lesions may be single or multiple, and they commonly affect the skull and proximal femora. Lung involvement is rare but carries a poor prognosis.

ANSWERS TO CASE HISTORIES

Case I

1. T4 estimation ★★★★
   T3 estimation ★★★★
   Blood cultures ★★
   Thyroid scan ★★
   Urinary porphyrins ★

2. Thyroid crisis ★★★★
   Acute intermittent porphyria ★
   Gross salt and water depletion ★
   Thyroid crisis (storm) is characterised by a fulminating increase in all the symptoms and signs of thyrotoxicosis: extreme irritability, delirium or coma, hyperpyrexia, tachycardia, hypotension, vomiting and diarrhoea. Treatment consists of rehydration, glucocorticoids, anti-thyroid medication, followed by oral/intravenous iodides.

Case II

1. Blood cultures ★★★★
   Ultrasound of liver ★★★★
   Radioisotope scan of liver ★★★★
   Stool microscopy and cultures ★★★★
   Amoeba complement fixation test ★★
   Pleural aspirate ★★
   Serum amylase ★★
   Coeliac arteriogram ★

2. Pyogenic liver abscess ★★★★
   Subphrenic abscess ★★
   Pancreatitis ★★
   Acute cholecystitis ★
   Hepatoma ★
   Blood cultures are positive in about 50% of cases of pyogenic liver abscess. The responsible organism reflects the source of infection; cholangitis is usually due to enteric organisms, particularly *E. coli*. Anaerobic streptococci (e.g. *Streptococcus melleri*) and bacteroides species are also frequent. Abscesses are more often multiple than solitary, and the right lobe is frequently involved. Pyogenic organisms reach the liver by the biliary system (cholangitis), the portal venous sytem (e.g. portal pyaemia from appendicitis), arterial blood (e.g. staphylococcal septicaemia), or by direct spread from contiguous structures (empyema of gall bladder, subphrenic abscess).

Case III

1. Edrophonium chloride ('Tensilon') test ★★★★
   Electromyography (EMG) ★★★★
   Antibodies for striated muscle, acetyl choline receptors ★★★★
   CT scan of the mediastinum ★★★★

2. Myasthenia gravis ★★★★
   Myasthenia gravis secondary to penicillamine therapy ★★★★
   The characteristic electromyographic feature of myasthenia gravis includes the onset of 'fatigue' on repetitive stimulation of a peripheral motor nerve. Thus, there is a decremental response of >10% from the first to the fifth response on maximal stimulation of a nerve to an involved muscle, at a frequency of 2–5 Hz.

Case IV

1. Screening of the diaphragms ★★★★
   Measurement of the transdiaphragmatic pressure ★★★★
   Transfer factor ★★★★
   Measurement of maximum inspiratory and expiratory pressures ★★★★
   Tensilon test ★★★★

2. Bilateral diaphragmatic weakness ★★★★

Case V

1. Blood gases ★★★★
   Electrocardiogram ★★★★
   Diuretic therapy ★★★★
   Urine culture ★★★★
   Echocardiogram ★★
   Blood cultures ★★
   Serum albumin ★★
   Creatinine clearance ★★
   ASO titre ★★
   Antinuclear factor ★★

2. Acute glomerulonephritis ★★★★
   Atrial septal defect ★★★★
   Biventricular failure ★★★★
   Hypertensive heart failure ★★★★

ANSWERS TO DATA INTERPRETATIONS

1. Atrial fibrillation ★★★★
   Left bundle branch block ★★★★
   Multifocal ventricular premature beats ★★★★
   Left axis deviation ★★★★

2. (a) Mitral stenosis ★★★★
   (b) Mitral incompetence ★★★★

Answers

3. Complete heart block with ventricular escape ★★★★

4. (a) Pyrophosphate arthropathy ★★★★
      Septic arthritis ★
   (b) X-ray of the joint ★★★★
      Culture of the joint fluid ★★
      Blood cultures ★★
      Rheumatoid factor 0

In 'pseudogout' there is usually a history of repeated gout-like attacks. The most commonly affected joints are the knees, symphysis pubis, hip and wrist joints, where calcification of cartilage may be found. Aspiration of synovial fluid during the acute attack will show calcium pyrophosphate dihydrate crystals, some of which are inside polymorphs.

5. Aortic stenosis ★★★★
   Hypertrophic obstructive cardiomyopathy ★★

The onset of symptoms in a patient with aortic stenosis is of great importance, as the subsequent course of the disease is downhill. In the symptomatic adult, surgery is indicated with significant narrowing of the valve ($<0.75 cm^2$), or a peak systolic gradient of 50mmHg.

6. (a) Double-stranded anti-DNA antibody ★★★★
      TPHA ★★★★
      C-reactive protein level ★★
      Hb$_S$ Ag ★★
      Complement levels ★
   (b) Systemic lupus erythematosus ★★★★
      Secondary syphilis ★★★★
      Viral infection ★★★★
      Rheumatoid arthritis ★★

False positive serological tests for syphilis may be 'acute' or 'chronic'. Acute (<6 months) false positive VDRL tests occur in atypical pneumonia, malaria, and bacterial and viral infections. Chronic false positive VDRL (>6 months) is common in SLE, narcotic addicts, leprosy, and in diseases associated with hyperglobulinaemia including rheumatoid arthritis, biliary cirrhosis, etc.

7. (a) Cytomegalovirus IgM antibody ★★★★
      Epstein-Barr IgM antibody ★★★★
      Paul-Bunnell test for heterophil antibodies ★★★★
      Isolation of CMV from urine ★★★★
      Complement fixation test for CMV ★★
      Reticulocyte count ★
   (b) Post-transfusional CMV infection ★★★★
      Epstein-Barr virus infection ★★
      Viral hepatitis ★★

CMV infection may occur after transfusion of infected blood. The incubation period after exposure is 30–60 days, and the illness lasts three to six weeks. Fever, myalgia, sore throat and rubelliform rash may occur. The haematological profile is identical to infectious mononucleosis, and transient production of the rheumatoid factor, cryoglobulins, ANF and cold agglutinins occur in both infections.

8. (a) Heinz body haemolytic anaemia ★★★★
      Haemolytic anaemia ★★
   (b) Salazopyrin treatment ★★★★

Although more typically seen in patients with glucose-6-phosphate-dehydrogenase deficiency, a Heinz body haemolytic anaemia with red cell fragmentation is occasionally seen in patients on salazopyrine, even with normal metabolism of red cell hexose monophosphate shunt. Haemoglobinaemia and haemoglobulinuria are usually of moderate degree and of limited duration, since only relatively old cells are vulnerable. Dapsone may also cause a similar haemolytic anaemia. Oxidative stresses leading to Heinz bodies occur through distinct steps:
(a) Inadequate NADPH with methaemoglobin formation;
(b) Oxidation of the thiol compound glutathione; (c) Oxidation of sulphydryl groups of haemoglobin, with denaturation and precipitation into Heinz bodies.

9. (a) Jejunal biopsy ★★★★
      Barium meal and follow-through ★★★★
      Faecal fat estimation ★★★★
      Plasma 1,25 dihydroxy-cholecalciferol level ★★★★
      Urinary calcium excretion ★★
      X-ray of pelvis (for pseudofractures) ★★
   (b) Malabsorption ★★★★
      Dietary Vitamin D and folic acid deficiency ★★
      Osteomalacia ★★

10. Acromegaly ★★★★
    Wilson's disease ★★★★
    Heroin abuse ★★★★
    Renal failure ★★★★

The paradoxical rise in growth hormone following a glucose tolerance test is not specific to acromegaly. where it occurs in 50–75% of cases.

Paper 11

Slide Interpretations

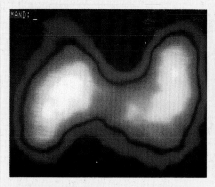
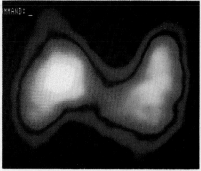
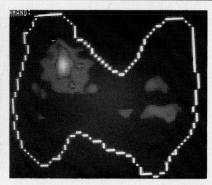

1. This is a MIBI/technetium subtraction scan. What is the diagnosis?

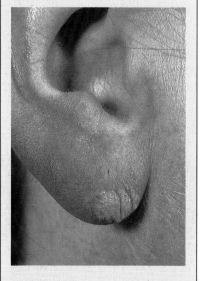

2. What is the diagnosis?

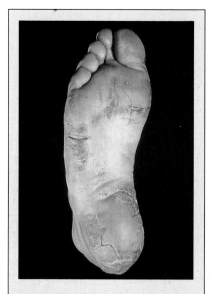

3. What is the diagnosis?

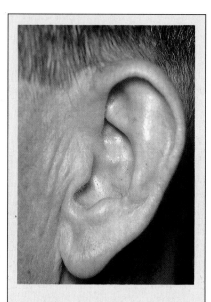

4. What is the diagnosis?

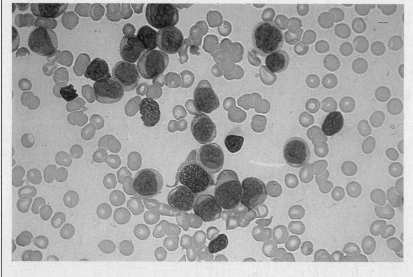

5. What diagnosis can be made from this blood film?

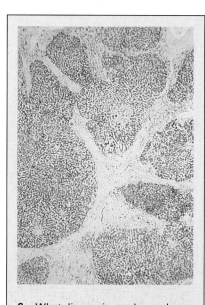

6. What diagnosis can be made from this liver biopsy?

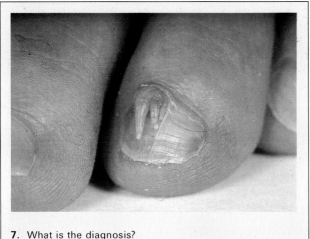

7. What is the diagnosis?

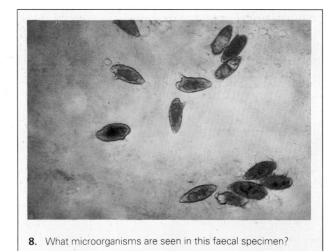

8. What microorganisms are seen in this faecal specimen?

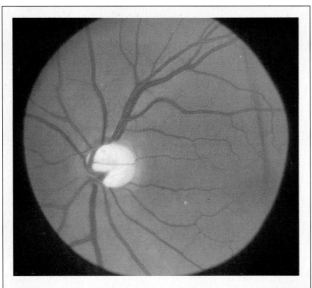

9. What is the most likely diagnosis?

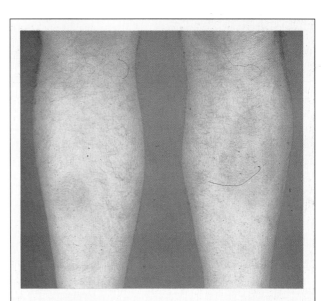

10. List a possible cause for these indurated, painless chronic lesions.

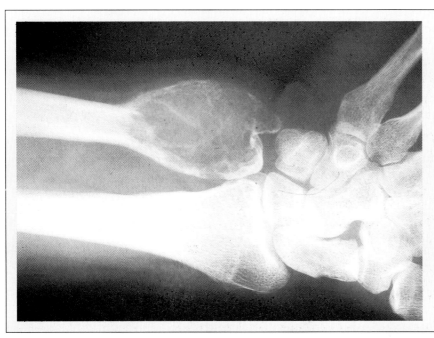

11. What is the diagnosis?

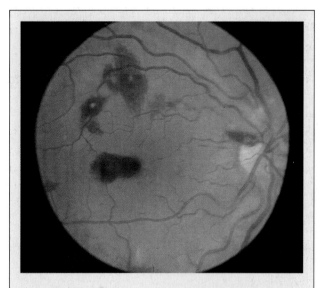

12. This fundal appearance was noted in a 45-year-old man under investigation for pyrexia of unknown origin.
What abnormality is shown?

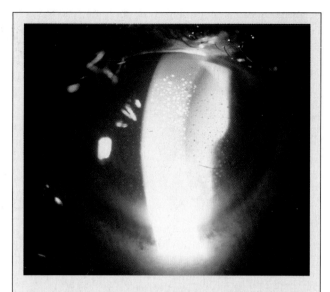

13. **(a)** What physical sign is demonstrated on this slit-lamp examination?
(b) Give two possible causes.

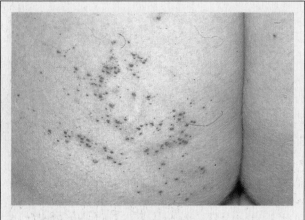

14. This patient was under treatment for a chronic renal condition.
What is the diagnosis?

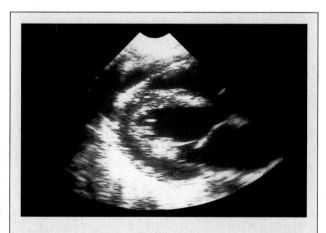

15. **(a)** What is the diagnosis?
(b) List four possible causes.

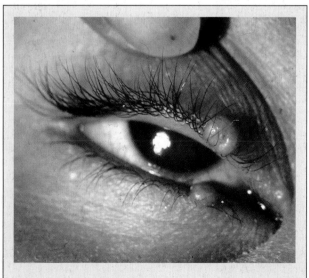

16. What is the diagnosis?

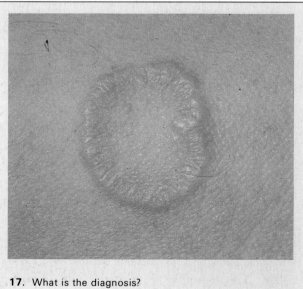

17. What is the diagnosis?

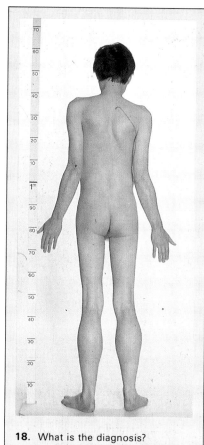

18. What is the diagnosis?

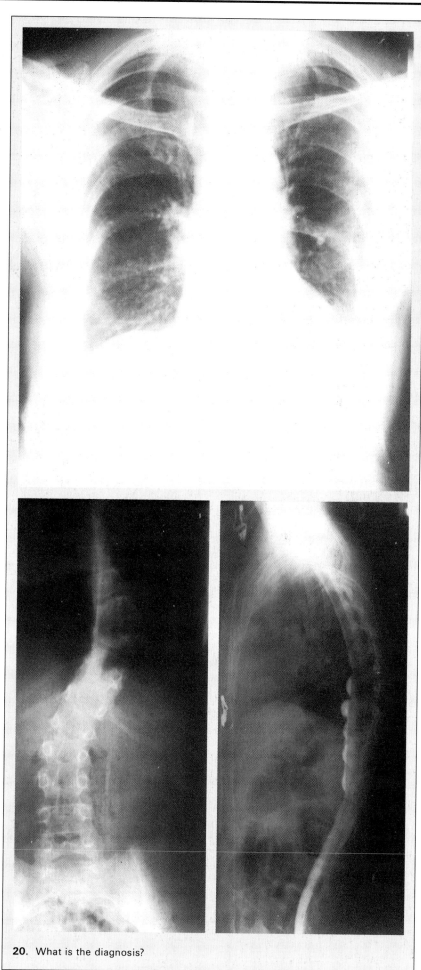

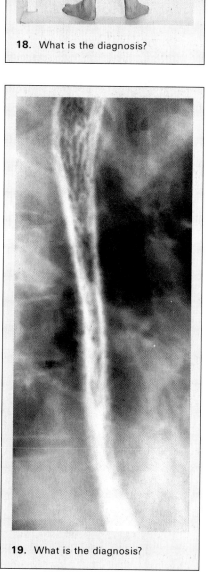

19. What is the diagnosis?

20. What is the diagnosis?

Case Histories

CASE I

A 42-year-old woman was perfectly well until six months earlier, when she began to experience headaches frequently associated with nausea and vomiting. She also complained of intermittent bouts of substernal heaviness lasting five to ten minutes, which were unrelated to exertion but sometimes precipitated by emotion. During the two months before admission, the patient was experiencing nausea and bouts of sweating. Recently, she had been suffering from occasional orthopnoea and nocturia up to twice nightly, with some ankle oedema. On the morning of admission, she was nauseous and vomited. In the afternoon, her husband, on returning home, found her cold and clammy and brought her into hospital. On questioning there was a ten-year history of mild hypertension controlled by hydrochlorothiazide, but with irregular compliance. She had also abused alcohol for many years, consuming up to half a bottle of spirits every night. She had smoked 40–60 cigarettes daily for over 30 years.

On examination her temperature was 37.8°C with a respiratory rate of 40/min. Pulse 120/min regular, blood pressure 180/120mmHg. The patient was clammy, agitated and dyspnoeic, and her limbs were mottled. Her jugulovenous pulse was raised by 3cm, and inspiratory crackles were heard over the lower two thirds of both lung fields. A fourth sound was present on auscultation. Abdominal examination disclosed a generalised distension with reduced bowel sounds and a tympanitic percussion note.

Investigations

HAEMATOLOGY
Hb: 16.4g/dl (16.4g/100ml); PCV: 0.54 (54%); WBC: 12 × 10⁹/l (12,000/mm³); Neutrophils: 93%; Band forms: 2%; Platelets: 480 × 10⁹/l (480,000/mm³); ESR: 21mm/h.

BIOCHEMISTRY
Urea: 7mmol/l (38mg/100ml); Creatinine: 180μmol/l (2.03mg/100ml); Glucose: 9.3mmol/l (167mg/100ml); Sodium: 138mmol/l (138mEq/l); Potassium: 3.5mmol/l (3.5mEq/l); Chloride: 99mmol/l (99mEq/l); Bicarbonate: 17mmol/l (17mEq/l); Serum glutamic oxaloacetic transaminase (SGOT): 149 iu/l; Serum amylase: 57SU; Arterial gases: pH:7.32; PaO₂: 7.2kPa (54mmHg); PaCO₂: 3.4kPa (26mmHg).

RADIOLOGY
ECG: Sinus tachycardia, QRS axis +60°; Roor R wave progression V₁ to V₃, non-specific ST segment abnormalities; CXR: Diffuse interstitial oedema; Prominent left ventricular border.

1. List three investigations which are warranted after her acute resuscitation.

2. What is the most likely underlying diagnosis?

CASE II

A 27-year-old woman was admitted to hospital for investigation of a rash. Over the past six months she had been prone to frequent attacks of cystitis, for which she was prescribed ampicillin. Three weeks before admission, she developed a white, irritant vaginal discharge for which an appropriate cream was prescribed. Shortly after commencing this treatment she developed severe dysuria and frequency, for which her GP prescribed cotrimoxazole. Five days later, the patient experienced a sudden onset of malaise, shivering, aches and pain in the muscles and joints, with a temperature of 39°C. During the ensuing hours she felt progressively worse, with increasing nausea, and she decided to stop the treatment. A violaceous rash appeared, and on the following day denuded areas had developed on her back.

On admission, the patient looked unwell, with a temperature of 40°C. She was uncomfortable on any movement. There was a diffuse symmetrical rash characterised by generalised, discrete and confluent erythematous areas that involved 85% of the skin surface. On her back, two flaccid bullae measuring 3 × 3cm were found. The epidermis seemed to slip over the deeper skin if traction was applied to it. The proximal two-thirds of the nailbeds were white, and the distal third was dark pink. Shotty lymph nodes were present in the axillae and inguinal region. Pulse was 120/min regular, blood pulse 95/60mmHg. The patient was dehydrated and her abdomen was generally tender.

Investigations

HAEMATOLOGY
Hb: 9g/dl (9g/100ml); PCV: 0.3 (30%); WBC: 3.0 × 10⁹/l (3,000/mm³); Neutrophils: 55%; Lymphocytes: 35%; Monocytes: 5%; Eosinophils: 5%; Platelets: 226 × 10⁹/l (226,000/mm³); ESR: 15mm/h.

BIOCHEMISTRY & RADIOLOGY
Urea and electrolytes: normal; Serum glutamic oxaloacetic transaminase (SGOT): 58iu/l; Lactic dehydrogenase: 301iu/l; Albumin: 33g/l (3.3g/100ml); Globulin: 40g/l (4.0g/100ml); Urinanalysis: normal; CXR: normal; ECG: normal.

1. Suggest three essential steps in this patient's management.

2. Suggest the most likely diagnosis.

CASE III

A 31-year-old man was admitted for investigation of a five-week history of pain in his lower lumbar region, associated with malaise. He had lost 6kg in weight. In the past, he had suffered from infective hepatitis at the age of 25, but had otherwise been well, having been declared medically fit on joining the army three years previously. Six months before admission, he was asked to leave the army when it was discovered that he was indulging in cannabis smoking. Three months previously, he had set out on a trip through Europe with a friend, which involved hitch-hiking and working sporadically on farms. The trip was interrupted by the onset of his illness.

On examination, he was febrile with a temperature of 37.4°C, and there was tenderness over the fifth lumbar and first sacral vertebrae. The movements of his back seemed to be limited by pain. Pulse 70/min regular, blood presure 120/80mmHg. There were no other abnormal findings on clinical examination.

Investigations

HAEMATOLOGY

Hb: 15.4g/dl (15.4g/100ml); WBC: 13 × 10⁹/l (13,000/
mm³); Neutrophils: 61%; Lymphocytes: 36%; Monocytes: 3%;
ESR: 88mm/h.

BIOCHEMISTRY & RADIOLOGY

Urea: 6.4mmol/l (39mg/100ml); Sodium: 136mmol/l
(136mEq/l); Potassium: 3.8mmol/l (3.8mEq/l); Bicarbonate:
23mmol/l (23mEq/l); Chloride: 103mmol/l (103mEq/l);
Bilirubin: 19μmol/l (1.1mg/100ml); Alkaline phosphatase:
110iu/l (14.3KAU/100ml); Calcium: 2.45mmol/l
(9.6mg/100ml); Phosphate: 1.08mmol/l (3.9mg/100ml);
SGOT: 53iu/l; Serum hydroxybutyrate dehydrogenase: 113iu/l;
Urinanalysis: normal; CXR: normal; X-ray of the lumbosacral
spine: irregularity of the right sacroiliac joint noted.

1. List three further diagnostically useful investigations.

2. Suggest the most likely diagnosis.

CASE IV

A 63-year-old farmer was admitted to hospital because of
weakness. He had been in good health previously, but eight days
prior to admission he developed symptoms of an upper
respiratory tract infection. Over the ensuing week the symptoms
gradually diminished, but he began to complain of aches in his
neck, back, thighs and calves, and noticed some numbness and
tingling in his fingers and toes. On the day of admission, he had
tried to get out of bed but found that his legs gave way. The
patient was only able to stand and walk with the support of his
wife. He was on no known medication, and denied any difficulty
with breathing, swallowing or urinating. There was no family
history of any significance.

On examination, the patient looked unwell and was
complaining of back pain. Pulse 78/min regular, blood pressure
110/70mmHg. The lungs were clear, abdominal examination
was normal, but the fauces were red. On neurological
examination, the fundi were normal. The patient was quite
unable to stand, and was only able to sit on the edge of the bed
with difficulty. Weakness of both distal and proximal musculature
was present, and deep tendon reflexes were absent. There was
loss of joint positional and vibration sense, and plantar responses
were flexor. Cranial nerve examination was unremarkable.

Investigations

Hb: 13.1g/dl (13.1g/100ml); MCV: 84fl (84/μm³); WBC:
13.6 × 10⁹/l (13,600/mm³); Band forms: 3%; ESR: 59mm/h;
Lumbar puncture: CSF pressure 80mm H₂O; Red cells:3/mm³;
Lymphocytes: 1/HPF; Glucose: 3.8mmol/l (68mg/100ml);
Protein: 0.8g/l (80mg/100ml).

1. List three diagnostically useful investigations

2. What is the most likely diagnosis?

CASE V

A 52-year-old man was referred following the onset of
generalised aches and pain associated with tingling and
numbness of the fingertips. He had been well until two weeks
previously, when he developed a generalised vesicular rash
thought to be chicken pox. Prior to this he had been in good
health, apart from mild essential hypertension for which he took
a beta-blocker. He drank five pints of beer and smoked 20
cigarettes daily. There was no family history of note.

On examination, he was pyrexial (37.8°C), his blood pressure
was 120/70mmHg, and pulse was 60/min regular. There were
no signs of meningeal irritation, and there was no papilloedema.
Mild bilateral ptosis was present, and the patient appeared
slightly dysarthric. Ataxia was present bilaterally on 'heel to toe'
testing. On the following day, the weakness of his arms and legs
was more marked. Examination of the cranial nerves revealed
mild external ophthalmoplegia. The deep tendon reflexes were
brisk, and gross limb and truncal ataxia was present. Twelve
hours later, he became drowsy and was noted to have an
irregular breathing pattern. In the evening of the second day of
hospitalisation, he became comatose with fixed dilated pupils
and absent oculocephalic, corneal, oculovestibular and gag
reflexes. In the morning his breathing seemed to improve and,
although still drowsy, he was rousable. Bilateral facial weakness
was noted.

Investigations

HAEMATOLOGY

Hb: 13.6g/dl (13.6g/100ml); MCV: 88fl (88μm³); WBC:
3.8 × 10⁹/l (3,800/mm³); ESR: 78mm/h.

BIOCHEMISTRY & SPECIAL INVESTIGATIONS

Urea: 5.4mmol/l (33mg/100ml); Creatinine: 0.08mmol/l
(0.94mg/100ml); Sodium: 134mmol/l (134mEq/l); Potassium:
4.6mmol/l (4.6mEq/l); Bicarbonate: 24mmol/l (24mEq/l);
Chloride: 100mmol/l (100mEq/l); Bilirubin: 16μmol/l
(0.98mg/100ml); Alkaline phosphatase: 76iu/l
(7.5KAU/100ml); Total protein: 74g/l (7.4g/100ml); Albumin:
39g/l (3.9g/100ml); SGOT: 33iu/l; Urinanalysis: no
abnormalities; Cerebrospinal fluid examination: Pressure:
180mm/H₂O; Cell content: 23 × 10⁶ lymphocytes/l (23/mm³);
Protein content: 0.63g/l (63mg/100ml); CSF glucose:
4.8mmol/l (84mg/100ml).

RADIOLOGY

CXR: normal cardiac size, no parenchymal shadowing of the
lungs; ECG: sinus rhythm, heart rate 54/min, normal QRS
amplitude; CT brain scan: no abnormalities seen.

1. List three investigations which would assist in the
patient's management at the time of admission.

2. What is the most likely diagnosis?

Data Interpretations

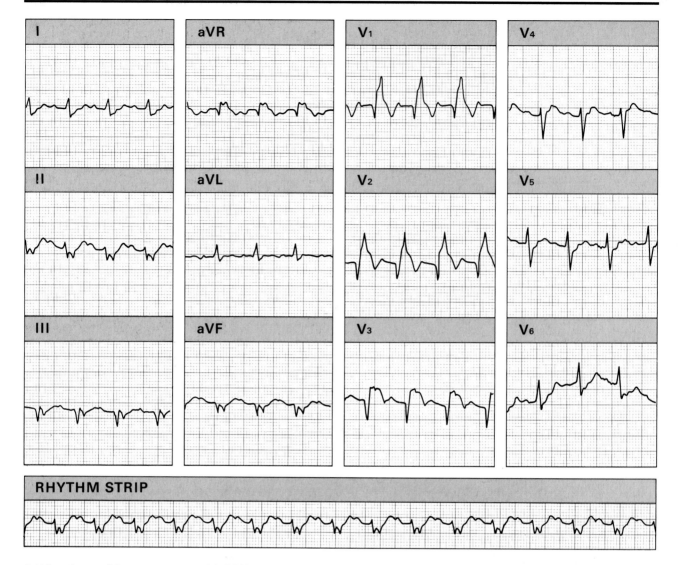

I	aVR	V₁	V₄
II	aVL	V₂	V₅
III	aVF	V₃	V₆

RHYTHM STRIP

1. What abnormalities are present on this ECG?

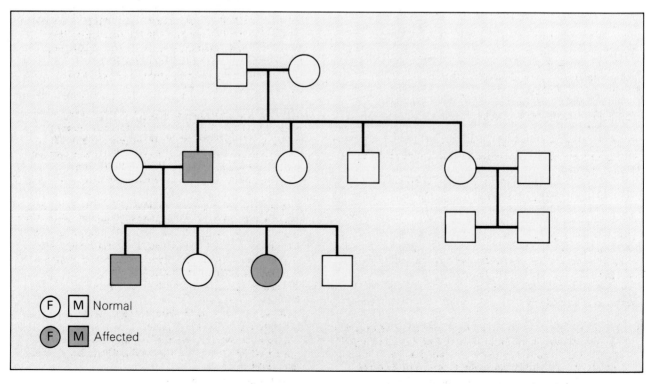

F ⃝ M ☐ Normal

Ⓕ ▣ Affected

11.8 2. (a) What mode of inheritance is illustrated in this family tree? **(b)** Give two examples of this type of inheritance.

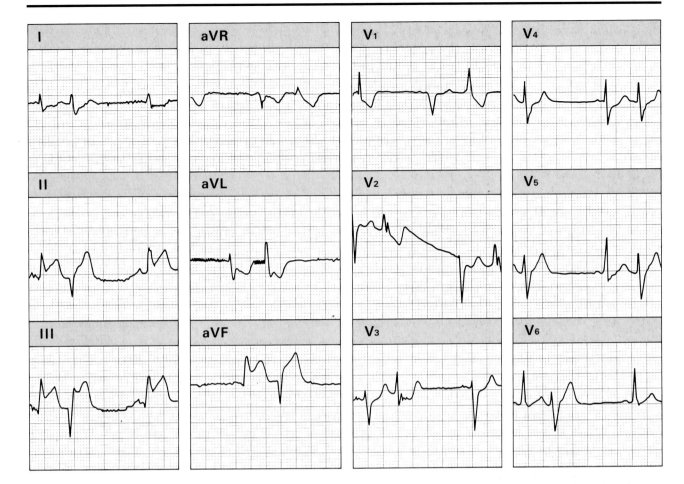

3. List two abnormalities on this electrocardiogram.

4. A 32-year-old woman is investigated because of polydipsia and polyuria. She undergoes a standard eight-hour water deprivation test, starting at 8.30am.

Time	Plasma Osmolality (mmol/kg)	Urine Osmolality (mmol/kg)
08.30	301	220
11.30	312	232
14.30	321	227
16.30	332	238

After $2\mu g$ intramuscular DDAVP at 16.30pm:

18.30	338	245

(a) What is the diagnosis?
(b) Suggest two possible causes.

5. A 67-year-old man was admitted following an episode of severe paroxysmal nocturnal dyspnoea. A cardiac catheter was performed.

	PRESSURES (mmHg)	
	Phasic	Mean
Right atrium	–	10
Right ventricle	60/0–12	–
Pulmonary artery	45–55/20	30
Pul Cap Wedge	–	30
Left ventricle	140/18–25	–
LVEDP	18–21	
Aorta	140/40	

What is the diagnosis?

6. A 3-month-old child is referred for investigation of recurrent seizures. On examination, the liver is found to be enlarged. Glucose: 2.1mmol/l (42mg/100ml); Bicarbonate: 14mmol/l (14mEq/l); pH: 7.30; Cholesterol: 14.6mmol/l (544mg/100ml); Triglycerides: 6.4mmol/l (480mg/100ml). What is the most likely diagnosis?

7. A 62-year-old man was investigated following an episode of amaurosis fugax. On examination, a mass was present in his left hypochondrium.
Hb: 14.6g/dl (14.6g/100ml); RCC: 8×10^{12}/l (8×10^6/mm³); PCV: 0.55 (55%); MCV: 68fl (68μm³); MCH: 18.5pg (18.5$\mu\mu$g); MCHC: 27g/dl (27g/100ml); WBC: 15.3×10^9/l (15,300/mm³); Neutrophils: 85%; Lymphocytes: 10%; Monocytes: 5%; Platelets: 475×10^9/l (475,000/mm³); Blood film: hypochromia ++, polychromasia +.
(a) List three diagnostically useful investigations.
(b) What is the diagnosis?

8. A 64-year-old woman gives a long history of tension headaches. She is now investigated for easy bruising.
PT: 15sec (control 13); PTTK: 46sec (control 36); TT: 12 sec (control 12); Bleeding time: 14.5 minutes (normal <8.5min); Platelets: 225×10^9/l (225,000/mm³).
Give one possible cause for the above findings.

9. A 44-year old man is investigated because of renal stones. Calcium: 2.97mmol/l (11.7mg/100ml); Albumin 38g/l (3.8 g/dl); PO_4: 1.22mmol/l (3.92mg/100ml); Urinary calcium excretion: 8.5mmol/24h; (340mg/24h). Following 10 days of 40mg oral hydrocortisone every eight hours, fasting calcium was 2.47mmol/l (9.7mg/100ml).
Suggest two possible causes for these findings.

10. A 64-year-old woman is investigated for ascites and unexplained pericardial effusion.
Sodium: 126mmol/l (126mEq/l); Cholesterol: 8.9mmol/l (345mg/100ml); CPK: 560 U/l; MCV: 98fl (98μm³); Blood film: 3% basophilia.
What is the likely diagnosis?

Answers

1. Right upper pole parathyroid adenoma ★★★★
   Hot thyroid nodule 0
   MIBI is taken up by both thyroid and parathyroid whereas technetium is taken up by the thyroid alone. If the images are subtracted, the parathyroid adenoma is revealed.

2. Gouty tophus ★★★★
   Polychondritis 0

3. Tylosis ★★★★
   Hyperkeratosis plantaris ★★
   This is diffuse plantar hyperkeratosis which is associated with hyperhydrosis and oesophageal carcinoma. There is hyperkeratotic thickening of the horny layer of the palms. The disorder is often familial.

4. Alkaptonuria ★★★★
   This rare condition leads to accumulation and urinary excretion of homogentisic acid. Fresh urine appears normal, but on standing the homogentisic acid becomes oxidized and imparts a characteristic black colour. The gradual deposition of homogentisic acid oxidation products in cartilage and in certain other tissues ultimately causes progressive tissue damage and disability. Pigmented oxidation products impart a bluish black colour to involved tissues that, together with the characteristic degenerative arthritis, results in the syndrome called ochronosis. Clinical features include bluish-black discolouration of sclerae and ears (as shown here), pigment deposits near the lateral rectus attachment sites in the sclerae, pigment deposits in the heart valves, larynx and tympanic membranes, darkening of the skin, and occasional pigmented renal or prostatic calculi.

5. Acute lymphoblastic leukaemia (ALL) ★★★★
   Acute myeloblastic leukaemia ★
   ALL has its highest incidence at 3–4 years of age, subsiding at 10 years. Bone tenderness, superficial lymphadenopathy, splenomegaly and hepatomegaly are common concomitants. A meningeal syndrome and testicular involvement are well-recognised. In ALL, blasts show no differentiation. Immunological markers and enzyme assays are useful in subdividing ALL into the common (non-B, non-T) variety (c-ALL), Thy-ALL (thymic cell origin), and the rare B-ALL. The enzyme TdT (terminal deoxynucleotidyl transferase) is raised in this condition.

6. Haemochromatosis with cirrhosis ★★★★

7. Periungal fibroma ★★★★
   Adenoma sebaceum ★★★★
   Epiloia ★★★★
   These lesions may affect fingers or toes, and are found in association with adenoma sebaceum in epiloia (tuberose sclerosis).

8. Schistosoma mansoni ★★★★
   Bilharzia ★★★★
   Man is the principal definitive host for *Schistosoma mansoni* and *S. japonicum*; the intermediate host is usually a snail of the genus *Biomphalaria*. The adult forms inhabit the portal and mesenteric veins, and female worms produce approximately 300 eggs every day. These are excreted in the faeces. (The eggs of *S. mansoni* seen in faeces characteristically show a lateral spine, as shown here). Infection is by fork-tailed cercariae. These penetrate human skin, lose their tails and migrate to the lungs and liver. On maturing they mate and migrate to their final habitat, where they may live for up to ten years.

9. Chronic glaucoma simplex ★★★★

Glaucoma ★★★★
Optic atrophy 0
There is complete attenuation of the retinal cup, together with extreme attenuation of the neuroretinal rim and undermining of its margin. There is also a nasal sweep of vessels.

10. Morphoea ★★★★
    Necrobiosis lipoidica ★

11. Giant cell tumour ★★★★
    Secondary deposits 0

12. Roth's spots ★★★★
    Vasculitis ★★
    There are haemorrhages with a white centre corresponding to a cotton wool spot (haemorrhagic infarct) or a collection of polymorphs. These may occur in SBE and SLE.

13. (a) Keratic precipitates ★★★★
    (b) Sarcoidosis ★★★★
        Syphilis ★★★★
        Still's disease ★★★★
    Cells in the anterior chamber agglutinate and circulate in the aqueous humour, to become deposited on the corneal endothelium. These 'keratic precipitates' constitute a classical feature of anterior uveitis, and are typically seen in the inferior quadrant of the cornea. This is probably due to the effect of gravity and convection currents within the aqueous humour.

14. Angiokeratoma corporis diffusum ★★★★
    Fabry's disease ★★★★
    Fordyce's disease 0
    This is a sex-linked disorder of sphingolipid metabolism, characterised by multiple angiokeratomas in the 'bathing trunk' area, intermittent pain in the fingers and toes from childhood onwards ('Fabry's crises'). This condition is also associated with hypohydrosis, corneal opacities and progressive renal disease. There is deficiency of α galactosidase-A activity in the plasma.

15. (a) Pericardial effusion ★★★★
        Cardiomyopathy 0
    (b) Tuberculosis ★★★★
        Coxsackie virus infection ★★★★
        Malignancy ★★★★
        Uraemia ★★★★
        Dressler's syndrome ★★★★
        Hypothyroidism ★★★★
        Connective tissue disease ★★★★

16. Molluscum contagiosum ★★★★
    Blepharitis 0
    Molluscum contagiosum produces characteristic clusters of pearly papules which become umbilicated as they grow. Lid margin involvement is common, as is a secondary follicular conjunctivitis, thought to be due to an immune reaction without direct conjunctival invasion by the oranism. 'Cheesy' contents, stained with haematoxylin, show characteristic 'molluscum bodies' (infected cytopathic epidermal cells). The condition is one cause of the Koebner phenomenon.

17. Granuloma annulare ★★★★
    Fungal infection (ringworm) 0
    The lesion starts as a nodule and slowly progresses to a spreading ring. Histologically, a dermal necrobiosis of collagen is seen. The hard, raised edge and absence of scaling and pruritus are usually sufficient to distinguish it from a fungal infection.

18. Becker's dystrophy ★★★★
    Duchenne muscular dystrophy ★★
    Becker's dystrophy has similar manifestations to Duchenne dystrophy, but the onset of the former is in late childhood or in

adolescence, with a slower progression of disease. Clinical similarities include pseudohypertrophy of the calf muscles (shown here), and increased serum creatine phosphokinase. Early weakness is proximal in the upper and lower limbs.

19. Oesophageal moniliasis ★★★★
    Oesophageal varices 0
    Oesophageal candidiasis causes substernal burning and either pain or a sensation of obstruction on swallowing.

20. Neurofibromatosis ★★★★
    Pott's disease of the spine 0
    Radiological features of neurofibromatosis include soft tissue fibromata, lung fibrosis, dumb bell tumours of the spinal cord, and bone dysplasia (e.g. 'ribbon' ribs) pseudoarthrosis and 'empty orbit' [absent sphenoid bone]).

ANSWERS TO CASE STUDIES

Case I

1. Cardiac enzymes ★★★★
   Daily electrocardiograms ★★★★
   Urinary VMA and metanephrines ★★★★
   Plasma catecholamine estimation ★★★★
   Abdominal CT scan ★★★★
   Meta-iodobenzylguanidine scan (MIBG) ★★★★
   Plain abdominal X-ray ★★

2. Phaeochromocytoma ★★★★
   Myocardial infarction ★★★★
   Renal infarction ★★
   Polyarteritis nodosa ★★
Acute medical crises associated with a phaeochromocytoma crisis (i.e. surge of catecholamine secretion) include myocardial infarction, stroke, acute renal failure and paralytic ileus.

Case II

1. Rehydration ★★★★
   Blood cultures ★★★★
   Skin biopsy ★★★★
   Urine cultures ★★
   ANF ★

2. Toxic epidermal necrolysis ★★★★
   Allergic reaction to sulphonamides ★★★★
   Staphylococcal scalded skin syndrome ★
   Toxic shock syndrome 0
   A large number of drugs have been implicated in the aetiology of toxic epidermal necrolysis. They include butazones, sulphonamides, phenolphthalein, pentazocine and ethambutol. It may also follow viral infections, measles immunisation, lymphoma and leukaemia, and graft-versus-host disease.

Case III

1. Blood cultures ★★★★
   Needle bone biopsy ★★★★
   Mantoux test ★★★★
   Radioisotope bone scan ★★★★
   CT scan of the sacroiliac region ★★

2. Pyogenic osteomyelitis ★★★★
   Tuberculous osteomyelitis ★★
   Extradural abscess ★★
   Ankylosing spondylitis ★★
   Malignant infiltration of sacroiliac area ★

Case IV

1. Nerve conduction studies ★★★★

Search for possible intoxication with manganese, mercury, lead ★★★★
Blood gases ★★★★
FVC, spirometry ★★★★
Paul Bunnell test ★★
Legionella titres ★★

2. Acute infective polyneuritis (Guillain-Barré syndrome)

Case V

1. Blood gases ★★★★
   Blood glucose ★★★★
   EEG ★★★★
   Magnetic resonance imaging of the brainstem ★★★★
   CSF virology (electron microscopy) ★★★★

2. Post-infectious brainstem encephalitis ★★★★
   Viral encephalitis ★★★★
   Wernicke's encephalopathy ★★
   Central pontine myelinolysis ★★
   Hepatic encephalopathy ★
   Drug intoxication ★
   Bacterial meningitis 0
   Cerebral lupus 0
   Subdural haematoma 0

ANSWERS TO DATA INTERPRETATIONS

1. Acute anteroseptal myocardial infarction ★★★★
   Left axis deviation ★★★★
   Old inferior infarction ★★★★
   First degree heart block ★★

2. (a) Autosomal recessive inheritance ★★★★
   (b) Cystic fibrosis ★★★★
       Wilson's disease ★★★★
       Homocystinuria ★★★★
       α_1 antitrypsin deficiency ★★★★

3. Acute inferior infarct ★★★★
   Bigeminus rhythm ★★★★

4. (a) Nephrogenic diabetes insipidus ★★★★
   (b) Hypercalcaemia ★★★★
       Hypokalaemia ★★★★
       Congenital ★★★★
       Lithium ★★★★
Nephrogenic diabetes insipidus may result from acquired renal disease, causing impairment of active chloride transport in the water-impermeable portion of the ascending loop of Henle; there is associated failure to establish a hypertonic environment in the medullary-collecting duct interstitium. The condition may also result from failure of the medullary-collecting duct to become water-permeable in the presence of vasopressin (VP). Drugs known to interfere with the action of VP include lithium, desmethylchlortetracycline and methoxyflurane. Hypokalaemia and hypercalcaemia act in part by antagonising the effects of VP on the collecting duct.

5. Aortic regurgitation ★★★★
   Left ventricular failure ★
   A left ventricular, end-diastolic pressure greater than 20mmHg suggests impairment of left ventricular function. Myocardial function is likely to be impaired and remain so after valve replacement, when the left ventricular end-diastolic diameter (by M mode echo) exceeds 55mm. Causes of aortic regurgitation include: rheumatic heart disease, subacute (or acute) bacterial endocarditis, ankylosing spondylitis, Marfan's syndrome, Hurler's syndrome,relapsing polychondritis and dissecting aortic aneurysm. **11.11**

Answers

6. Glycogen storage disease (Type I) ★★★★
Hypoglycaemia is common and rapid in onset with fasting. A
metabolic acidosis is the rule.

7. (a) Red cell mass/plasma volume ★★★★
LAP score ★★★★
Fe and TIBC estimation ★★★★
Bone marrow examination ★★★★
IVU ★
PaO_2 ★
Uric acid level ★
Serum B12 binding capacity ★

(b) Polycythaemia rubra vera (PRV) with iron deficiency ★★★★
PRV ★★
Characteristic laboratory findings in PRV are:
Raised haemoglobin, haematocrit and red cell count;
Neutrophil leucocytosis (in 50% of cases) — some have raised
basophils and platelets (50%);
Raised neutrophil alkaline phosphatase score;
Raised serum B12 binding capacity;
Hypercellular marrow with prominent megacaryocytes.

8. Salicylate consumption ★★★★
Heparin therapy 0

9. Malignancy-associated hypercalcaemia ★★★★
Sarcoidosis ★★★★
Hypervitaminosis D ★★★★
Thyrotoxicosis ★★★★
Non-suppression of calcium in serum following a ten-day course
of hydrocortisone (40mg eight-hourly) is consistent with primary
hyperparathyroidism. About 50% of tumour-associated
hypercalcaemia fails to suppress with glucocorticoids. All other
causes of hypercalcaemia suppress with glucocorticoids.

10. Hypothyroidism ★★★★
Systemic lupus erythematosus ★
Disseminated tuberculosis ★
Clinically discernible ascites with myxoedema usually occurs in
association with pleural and pericardial effusions. Like effusions
into the other serous cavities, the ascitic fluid is rich in protein
and mucopolysaccharides. Basophilia, hyponatraemia
(inappropriate ADH secretion) and raised creatine phosphokinase
are well-recognised abnormalities in severe hypothyroidism.

Paper 12

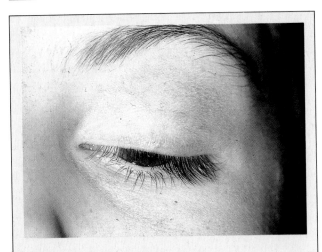

1. What is the likely cause of this appearance?

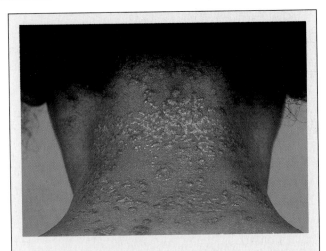

2. What is the likely cause of this chronic, non-pruritic eruption in this West Indian girl?

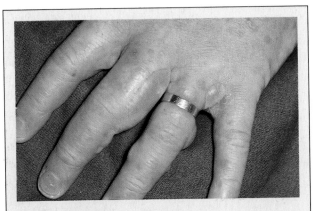

3. This pruritic and bullous eruption had been present for eight weeks on the hands of a 36-year-old woman, in the third trimester of pregnancy. What is the diagnosis?

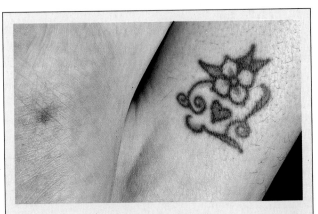

4. These are the cutaneous appearances of a 35-year-old patient, a known drug addict. She was suffering from a PUO. What is the diagnosis?

5. What is the most likely cause of these appearances?

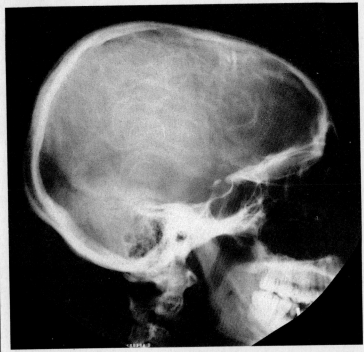

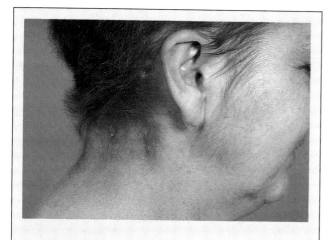

6. List two possible causes to account for this appearance of recent onset in a 67-year-old woman.

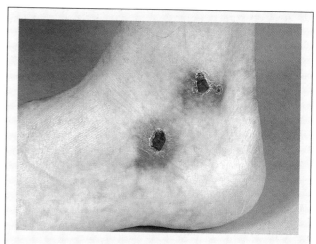

7. These ulcers were chronic and very tender. What is the most likely diagnosis?

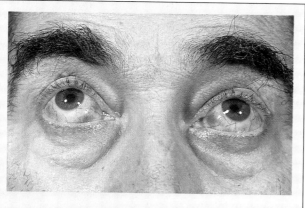

8. These are the eyes of a patient with a long-standing joint complaint. What abnormality is shown?

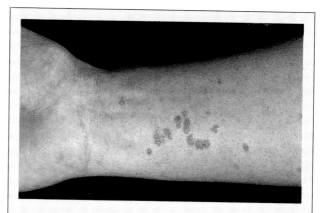

9. What is the diagnosis?

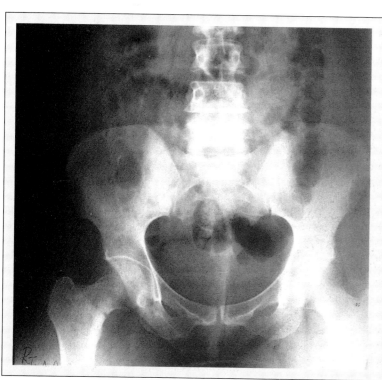

10. This abdominal radiograph is taken from a 46 year old Indian woman with malabsorption. Recently she has had difficulty standing from the sitting position.
What abnormality is shown?

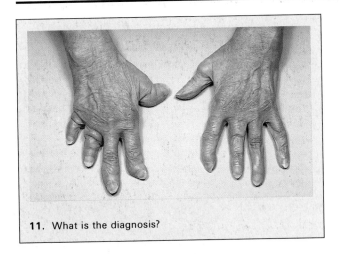

11. What is the diagnosis?

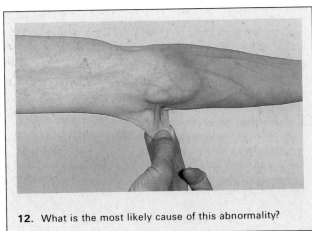

12. What is the most likely cause of this abnormality?

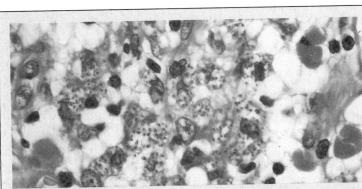

13. This bone marrow aspirate was taken from a patient with a pyrexia of unknown origin and splenomegaly.
What is the diagnosis?

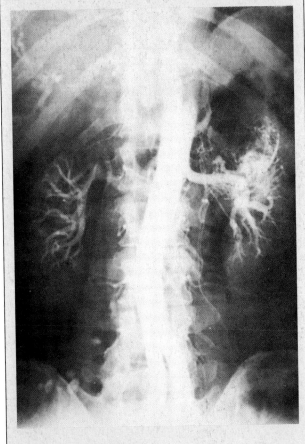

14. What is the diagnosis?

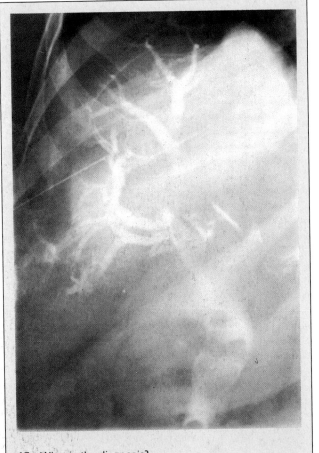

15. What is the diagnosis?

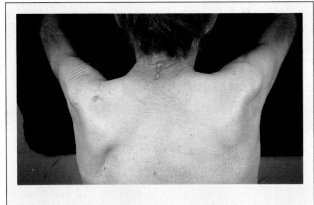

16. What single diagnosis would explain this appearance?

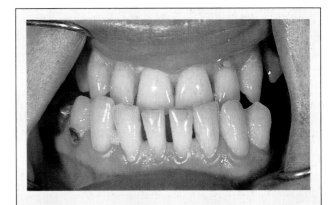

17. What is the diagnosis?

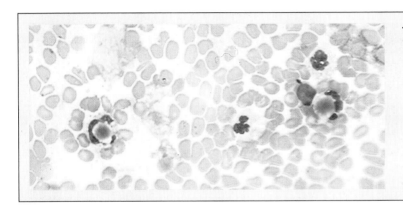

18. Give two possible causes for the phenomenon demonstrated on this blood film.

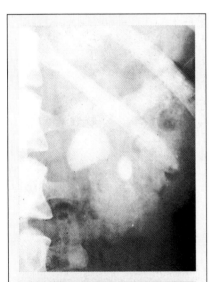

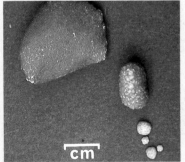

19. What is the probable nature of these renal stones?

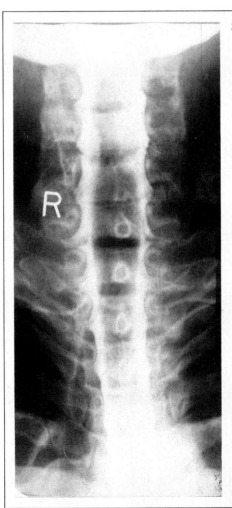

20. This 20-year-old girl presented with wasting of the hands. A cervical myelogram was performed. What is the most likely diagnosis?

Case Histories

CASE I

A 48-year-old man was admitted for investigation of clumsiness. He had been well until 18 months before, when he gradually developed mild incoordination and slurring of speech. After two months this seemed to improve, but three months later his speech once again became slow and hesitant, and he was admitted for investigations, where examination revealed mild dysarthria, horizontal nystagmus on lateral gaze, and prominent dysmetria with intention tremor on 'finger to nose' testing. The gait was wide-based, and the patient lurched unpredictably in walking. Following a CT scan of the brain, he was given a course of ACTH, although without beneficial effect. After discharge from hospital, his course gradually deteriorated, and he became unable to walk alone without falling. Shaking of the arms was severe when he attempted to support himself. He became confused, and developed incontinence of urine.

On admission, the patient's speech was fragmented and he used paraphrasic expressions. He was disorientated in time and place. Cranial nerves were normal and muscle strength was preserved. The tendon reflexes were brisk, and the right plantar reflex was equivocal. Hoffmann, grasp and rooting reflexes were present bilaterally. There were numerous myoclonic twitches of the face. The rest of the clinical examination was unremarkable.

1. List three essential investigations.

2. What is the most likely diagnosis?

CASE II

A 34-year-old nurse was admitted to hospital with a seven-day history of vulval pain and low back discomfort. Two days previously she had developed dysuria. On the day prior to admission, she developed a temperature of 38°C, with headache and severe backache, some neck stiffness, vomiting and photophobia. She was on oral contraceptives. She complained of a vaginal discharge, whitish in colouration, which had been present for five days.

On examination, she appeared drowsy but rousable. Temperature was 37.9°C. Examination of the head and neck was unremarkable, and lungs appeared clear. Pulse 122/min regular, blood pressure 130/80mmHg. The abdomen was normal. Examination of the vulva revealed excoriations and tenderness during palpation in the parametrial areas and posteriorly. She had moderate neck stiffness, and Kernig's sign was positive. Neurological examination was otherwise unremarkable.

Investigations

Hb: 11.6g/dl (11.6g/100ml); WBC: 6.4 × 10⁹/l (6,400/mm³); Neutrophils: 54%; ESR: 40mm/h; Urine electrolytes: normal; CXR: clear; Urinalysis: Proteinuria positive on albustix; CSF examination; White cells: 750 × 10⁶/l (750/mm³), predominantly mononuclear cells; Protein: 1.8g/l (180mg/100ml); Glucose: 4.6mmol/l (83mg/100ml); Simultaneous blood glucose: 6.1mmol/l (110mg/100ml); Culture of CSF: negative.

1. List three investigations which would assist in the management of this patient.

2. Suggest the most likely diagnosis.

CASE III

A 35-year-old woman was admitted to hospital for investigation of postpartum jaundice associated with pruritus. Eight weeks previously, she had delivered a healthy boy after an uncomplicated pregnancy. The jaundice had appeared gradually five weeks later, and it was not associated with any other constitutional symptoms. In her history, apparently several people had commented that she occasionally looked 'yellow' for periods lasting two to three weeks. This was sometimes associated with itching. However, at no time had she passed dark urine or pale stools. Following her first pregnancy five years previously, she had developed mild hypertension for which she was receiving a thiazide diurectic. This was continued during her most recent pregnancy. She did not drink excessive quantities of alcohol, and was a non-smoker. Systemic enquiries were otherwise unremarkable.

On examination, the patient was clearly icteric but with no features of chronic liver disease. There was no lymphadenopathy, and examination of the abdomen revealed no evidence of hepato- or splenomegaly. Pelvic examination was unremarkable. The rest of the examination was normal.

Investigations

HAEMATOLOGY
Hb: 11.5g/dl (11.5g/100ml); MCV: 86fl (86µm³); WBC: 9.5 × 10⁹/l (9,5000/mm³); Normal differential count; ESR: 18mm/h.

BIOCHEMISTRY & RADIOLOGY
Urea and electrolytes: normal; Bilirubin: 55µmol/l (3.23mg/100ml); Alkaline phosphatase: 86iu/l (11.5KAU/100ml); Total protein: 68g/l (6.8g/100ml); Albumin: 36g/l (3.6g/100ml); Calcium: 2.5mmol/l (9.69mg/100ml); Serum glutamic oxaloacetic transaminase (SGOT): 44iu/l; Serum hydroxybutyrate dehydrogenase: 112iu/l; Urinalysis: bile +++; CXR: normal.

1. List three investigations which would assist in establishing the diagnosis.

2. What is the most likely diagnosis?

A 68-year old woman was admitted for investigation of recurrent right basal pneumonia. She had been well until three months previously when, following a flu-like illness, she developed fever associated with rigors and some coughing. However, there was no sputum production or chest pain. She was seen by her GP who elicited physical signs of early consolidation in the right mid and low zones. She was prescribed oral cephradine therapy, following which she appeared to improve. A chest X-ray, carried out two weeks later, showed some increased lung markings in the right lower zone, but it was otherwise normal. However, her symptoms recurred subsequently, and a week later she again developed rigors with a dry cough. In the past she had been well, except for arthritis affecting her distal interphalangeal joints and the base of her right thumb. She had had both tonsils and her adenoids removed as a child, and an appendicectomy at the age of 31. She was a spinster and had looked after her frail father who died of tuberculosis at the age of 91. She had smoked 10 cigarettes a day for 30 years. Prior to admission, she had lost 2kg in weight. Her general health had otherwise been good, except for a chronic nasal dryness for which she used regular nose drops with good effect.

On examination her temperature was 39°C, with a pulse of 105/min and a blood pressure of 120/70mmHg. She was tachypnoeic with mild peripheral cyanosis. There was no lymphadenopathy, and cardiac auscultation was unremarkable. Examination of the chest revealed dullness at the right lung base with bronchial breathing and some aegophony. Crackles were audible at the left mid and low zones. The abdomen was normal and examination of the central nervous system unremarkable.

Investigations

HAEMATOLOGY
Hb: 11.1g/dl (11.1g/100ml); PCV: 0.36 (36%); WBC: 16.5 × 10⁹/l (16,500/mm³); Neutrophils: 84%; ESR: 104mm/h.

BIOCHEMISTRY & RADIOLOGY
Urea: 3.8mmol/l (23mg/100ml); Electrolytes: normal; Glucose: 6.4mmol/l (115mg/100ml); Globulin: 36g/l (3.6g/100ml); Albumin: 34g/l (3.4g/100ml); Arterial gases: PaO_2: 8.1kPa (61mmHg); $PaCO_2$: 4.2kPa (32mmHg; pH: 7.45; Mantoux test: 1/1000 negative; CXR: shallow inspiration, consolidation of the right lower and middle lobes noted. Calcific scarring visible in the right apex. Very patchy consolidation of the left lower zone.

1. List two investigations which would be diagnostically useful.

2. List two possible diagnoses.

A 34-year-old accountant was found to be hypokalaemic following a routine set of blood tests as part of an insurance examination, and was therefore referred for further investigations. His past medical history had been totally unremarkable, except for two episodes in his twenties of sudden onset of thirst and urinary frequency. On each occasion, he had been seen by his GP who had failed to find any glucose in his urine. Since these episodes had resolved spontaneously, he had not pursued the medical investigations further. Three months prior to his insurance examination, he had suffered a further incident, becoming extremely weak and generally feeling lethargic. Otherwise he was well, and took no medication or laxatives. In his family history, however, an uncle had also undergone intensive investigations for a low potassium. Systemic enquiry showed no abnormal symptoms, except for occasional paraesthesiae in his fingers.

On examination, he was a well-looking man, with a pulse of 66/min regular and a blood pressure of 130/80mmHg. Heart and lungs were normal, as were the cranial nerves. There was nothing of note in the abdomen; the kidneys were not palpable. Dip-stick urinanalysis was normal.

Investigations

HAEMATOLOGY
Hb: 14.6g/l (14.6g/100ml); PCV: 0.51 (51%); MCV: 85fl (85μm³); WBC: 6.8 × 10⁹/l (6,800/mm³); Normal differential count; ESR: 12mm/h.

BIOCHEMISTRY & RADIOLOGY
Sodium: 135mmol/l (135mEq/l); Potassium: 3mmol/l (3mEq/l); Chloride: 88mmol/l (88mEq/l); Bicarbonate: 35mmol/l (35mEq/l); SGOT: 37iu/l; Bilirubin: 12μmol/l (0.7mg/100ml); Total protein: 68g/l (6.8g/100ml); Albumin: 39g/l (3.9g/100ml); Calcium: 2.38mmol/l; Phosphate: 0.72mmol/l; Magnesium: 0.75mmol/l (1.5mEq/l); Lying aldosterone: 556pmol/l; CXR: normal.

1. List two diagnostically useful investigations.

2. What is the most likely diagnosis?

Data Interpretations

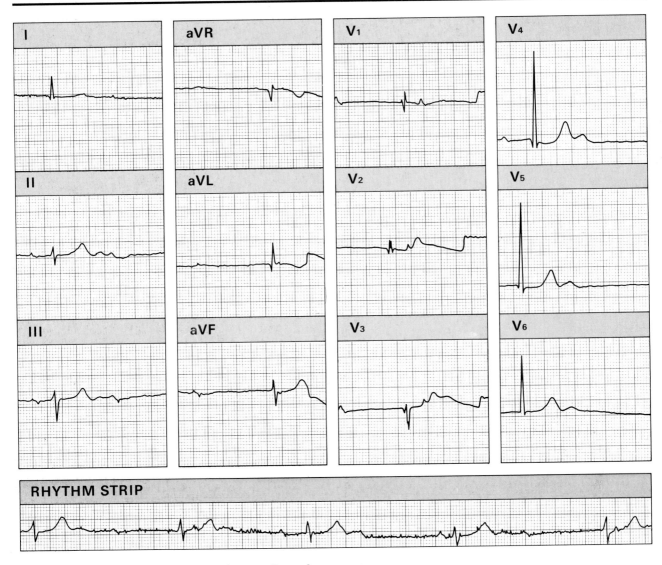

I	aVR	V₁	V₄
II	aVL	V₂	V₅
III	aVF	V₃	V₆

RHYTHM STRIP

1. What abnormalities are present on this electrocardiogram?

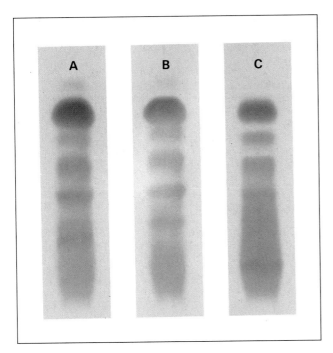

A   B   C

2. **A** and **B** represent the electrophoretic strips from normal plasma and serum respectively. **C** is taken from a patient. What is the most likely diagnosis in **C**?

3. An 18-year-old woman is admitted for investigation of recent onset of generalised weakness and diplopia. She had recently had a mild attack of influenza.
Peak flow rate: 210/min (predicted 390–500); FEV₁: 1.6/l; FVC: 2.1/l; PaO₂: 10.1kPa (76mmHg); PaCO₂: 6.7kPa (50mmHg).
(a) What two investigations are urgently required?
(b) What abnormality is present?

4. A 65-year-old woman gave a two-month history of lower sternal dysphagia and a two stone weight loss. An eruption had appeared on the back of her hands, and her face had become swollen.
Hb: 11.4g/dl (11.4g/100ml); MCV: 82fl (82μm³); WBC: 7.4 × 10⁹/l (7,400/mm³); Platelets: 655 × 10⁹/l (655,000/mm³); ESR: 21mm/h; SGOT: 124iu/l; CPK: 504iu/l.
(a) List two essential investigations.
(b) What is the most likely diagnosis?

5. A 28-year-old woman is investigated because of anaemia.
Hb:8.6g/dl (8.6g/100ml); MCV: 110fl (110μm³); WBC: 8.2 × 10⁹/l (8,200/mm³); Platelets: 202 × 10⁹/l (202,000/mm³); Reticulocytes: 1.6%; Hydroxybutyrate dehydrogenase (HBD): 1,260U/l.
A deoxyuridine suppression test is carried out on her bone marrow (BM): BM + dU = 41% BM + B12 = 40% BM + Folic acid = 10%.
(a) Suggest two diagnostically useful investigations.
(b) What is the diagnosis?

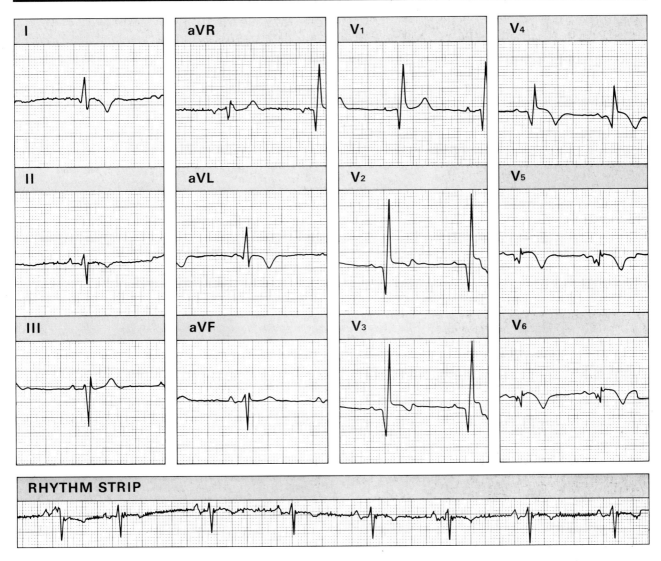

I	aVR	V1	V4
II	aVL	V2	V5
III	aVF	V3	V6

RHYTHM STRIP

6. What abnormalities are shown on this electrocardiogram?

7. A 63-year-old woman was investigated because of muscular pain and weakness.
   Hb: 9.6g/dl (9.6g/100ml); MCV: 98fl (98μm³); Calcium: 1.88mmol/l (7.39mg/100ml); Phosphate: 0.66mmol/l (2.12mg/100ml); Alkaline phosphatase: 146iu/l; Albumin: 31g/l (3.1g/100ml).
   (a) List four essential follow-up investigations.
   (b) What single diagnosis would explain the above findings?

8. A 16-year-old girl is receiving chemotherapy for a high-grade lymphoma. She becomes septicaemic and is treated with gentamicin. Within three days, she complains of paraesthesiae and has a convulsion.
   Glucose: 3.1mmol/l (56mg/100ml); Sodium: 128mmol/l (128mEq/l); Calcium: 1.66mmol/l 6.5mg/100ml); Phosphate: 0.65mmol/l (2.1mg/100ml); Magnesium: 0.43mmol/l; Glycosuria: +.
   (a) What is the most likely diagnosis?
   (b) What is the indicated treatment?

9. A 14-year old girl is investigated for persistent jaundice following an episode of infective hepatitis four months previously. She now complains of pain in the right hypochondrium and nausea.
   Hb: 13.4g/dl (13.4g/100ml); Bilirubin: 55μmol/l (3.2mg/100ml); Alkaline phosphatase: 154iu/l; Urobilinogen: +; Bilirubinuria: negative.
   (a) What is the most likely diagnosis?
   (b) Suggest two confirmatory investigations.

10. A 56-year-old West Indian woman was admitted following a three-day history of dysuria and urinary frequency. On examination, she was pyrexial (39°C), drowsy and severely dehydrated.
    Hb: 16.2g/dl (16.2g/100ml); WBC: 19.6 × 10⁹/l (19,600/mm³); Neutrophils: 91%; Sodium: 160mmol/l (160mEq/l); Potassium: 5.2mmol/l (5.2 mEq/l); Chloride: 128mmol/l (128mEq/l); Bicarbonate: 23mmol/l (23mEq/l); Urea: 31mmol/l (188mg/100ml); Urine: pus cells +++; Glucose: 5%; Ketones: negative.
    (a) Suggest two essential investigations.
    (b) What is the likely diagnosis?

Answers

1. Dermatomyositis ★★★★
   Orbital cellulitis ★
   The magenta ('heliotrope') colour, with oedema affecting particularly the upper lid, is virtually pathognomonic. Malignant disease is reported to be present in up to 25% of adult cases. Other cutaneous manifestations include nailfold telangiectasia, with vascular thromboses, scarring and ragged cuticles, and a rash over the dorsum of the knuckles.

2. Cutaneous sarcoidosis ★★★★
   Molluscum contagiosum 0
   Tuberculosis 0
   Sarcoidosis produces papules, nodules or plaques in the skin in nearly 50% of cases. Lesions may be of any shape; in the Caucasian, they are usually reddish brown and vary in number from one to more than a hundred. The surface of the skin is unchanged and the granulomatous infiltrate can be sensed by palpation. The commonest sites are the face, neck and back of the arms.

3. Herpes gestationatis ★★★★
   Pemphigoid ★
   Drug reaction ★
   Urticaria 0
   The lesions typically consist of pruritic blisters and plaques resembling urticaria. The eruption usually occurs from the fifth month of pregnancy to the early post-partum period. It is best regarded as a form of pemphigoid occurring during pregnancy, which resolves after parturition but may recur with further pregnancies.

4. Janeway lesion ★★★★
   Subacute bacterial endocarditis ★★★★
   Janeway lesions are haemorrhagic, macular, flat, painless plaques with a predilection for the palms and the soles. They are most commonly found in patients with acute staphylococcal endocarditis and are frequently multiple. Cutaneous manifestations of endocarditis (found in about 50% of patients) include petechiae, (in the conjunctiva, palate, buccal mucosa, and extremities), Osler's nodes, Roth's spots, splinter haemorrhages and clubbing of the nails.

5. Sturge–Weber syndrome ★★★★
   Characteristically, the skull X-ray shows serpiginous (leptomeningeal) calcifications located in the brain parenchyma, underlying the vascular malformation of the pia mater. These intracranial calcifications are first seen on CT scan but become evident on plain skull films by the end of the second decade. Other cardinal features are: the vascular naevus (port-wine stain); and seizures (in 90% of cases), which usually begin in the first year of life.

6. Internal malignancy ★★★★
   Drug therapy with minoxidil ★★★★
   Drug therapy with cyclosporin ★★★★
   Drug therapy with diazoxide ★★★★
   Hypertrichosis languinosa consists of long, fine, silky hair on the face and other sites normally clinically hairless (it does not involve palms and soles). It is associated with malignancy in the bronchus, gall bladder; rectum and bladder.

7. Polyarteritis nodosa ★★★★
   Trauma ★
   Livedo reticularis and chronic painful ulceration suggest polyarteritis nodosa.

8. Scleromalacia ★★★★
   Ochronosis ★★
   Osteogenesis imperfecta 0

This is scleromalacia, a form of scleritis which results in devitalisation and sloughing of scleral tissue. There is progressive thinning of the sclera in the absence of symptoms and without inflammation, as a result of arteriolar occlusion in the deep vascular network. It is nearly always associated with severe long-standing rheumatoid arthritis.

9. Lichen planus ★★★★
   This highly pruritic eruption consists of flat-topped papules, polygonal, shiny, violaceous and slightly scaly in appearance. Note the white lacy pattern (Wickham's striae) on the surface of some the lesions. The characteristic histological features are: (a) Focal thickening of the granular layer (hypergranulosis) and irregular thickening of the malpighian layer (acanthosis); (b) Upper dermal mononuclear infiltrate, extending to the dermoepidermal junction; (c) Dermal papilla broadening and rete ridge narrowing.

10. Looser's zone (pseudofracture) of right femoral neck ★★★★
    Fracture of the right femoral neck ★
    This is the diagnostic radiological feature of osteomalacia.

11. Psoriatic arthropathy ★★★★
    Arthritis mutilans ★★★★
    Osteoarthritis 0
    Rheumatoid arthritis 0
    Three patterns of arthritis occur in association with psoriasis: (a) An insidious polyarthritis affecting the distal interphalangeal joints and the sacroiliacs. Nail changes are common; (b) In 'arthritis mutilans' there is a deforming arthritis in which erosions and bone resorption is marked. Radiologically, there is 'telescoping' of the phalanges and the 'opera glass' hand. The cervical spine, hips and S.I. joints are frequently involved; (c) Psoriatic arthritis may occur in a form indistinguishable from seronegative rheumatoid arthritis. Rarely, psoriatic arthritis may occur as an acute monoarticular arthritis.

12. Ehlers-Danlos syndrome ★★★★
    Cutis laxa ★★★★
    There is hyperextensible skin which, with hyperextensive joints, is highly suggestive of Ehlers-Danlos synbdrome. In cutis laxa the skin is also hyperextensible, but in contrast it is loose and inelastic, hanging in folds; joint hypermobility is not usually present. Hyperelastic skin may also be found in Bonnevie-Ullrich-Turner syndrome, but other features of this disorder (dwarfism, webbing of the neck, gonadal dysgenesis and XO karyotype) establish the diagnosis.

13. Leishmaniasis ★★★★
    Kala-azar ★★★★
    In the diagnosis of kala-azar, Leishman-Donovan bodies may be present in large mononuclear cells or in bone marrow macrophages. The parasites (amastigotes) are seen as round or oval bodies, 2–5 μm in diameter, containing a large round or oval-looking nucleus, and a smaller, more deeply stained and usually rod-shaped kinetoplast.

14. Right renal artery stenosis (RAS) ★★★★
    Polycystic kidneys 0
    Renovascular hypertension accounts for 5% of hypertension cases. The commonest cause of RAS is atheroma (60%), followed by fibromuscular hyperplasia (35%). There is an increased incidence of RAS with neurofibromatosis, and of cerebral aneurysm with fibromuscular hyperplasia.

15. Gall stones in the common bile duct ★★★★
    Biliary obstruction ★★
    This contrast radiograph illustrates the technique of percutaneous transhepatic cholangiography; this is used in cases of obstructive jaundice where ultrasound has shown the presence of dilated ducts. Like endoscopic retrograde

cholangiopancreatography, it will yield valuable anatomical information as to the site of the obstruction. Biliary peritonitis is the major complication.

16. Herpes zoster infection ★★★★
    Serratus anterior weakness ★★
    Winging of the left scapula ★
    Herpes zoster is not infrequently associated with a peripheral mononeuritis or local encephalomyelitis, which may cause muscle paralysis and atrophy in the area of the segmental rash. Here, the long thoracic nerve ($C_{5,6,7}$) has been affected. Other major neurological manifestations of herpes zoster include transverse or ascending myelitis, disseminated encephalitis and acute cerebellar ataxia.

17. Acromegaly ★★★★
    Prognathism ★
    Malocclusion ★
    There is obvious prognathism and separation of the teeth due to bony and soft tissue overgrowth.

18. Systemic lupus erythematosus ★★★★
    Chronic active hepatitis ★★★★
    Lymphoma ★★
    Dermatomyositis ★
    Rheumatoid arthritis ★
    Sjogren's disease ★
    The film demonstrates the 'LE cell' phenomenon. The LE cell factor is IgG antibody (Ab) to native DNA. LE cell formation is an *in vitro* event; the *in vivo* counterpart is the haematoxylin body in tissues. The test is performed in two stages: First, the Ab is incubated with a source of dead cell nuclei, which allows it to bind to the nucleoprotein. Next, living polymorphs are added, and in the presence of complement they phagocytose the nuclei with fixed Ab. Lysosomal enzymes react on the nucleus causing denaturation of proteins, with swelling, loss of chromatin pattern and change in staining properties. On staining, LE cells are seen as polymorphs containing a large, homogeneous, purplish staining inclusion. The LE cell is positive in 75% of SLE cases.

19. Cystine stones ★★★★
    Hyperoxaluria ★★
    Calcium oxalate stones ★
    Calcium phosphate/magnesium ammonium phosphate ★
    Urate stones 0
    Xanthine stones 0
    Cystinuria is characterised by deficient transport of dibasic aminoacids, cystine, lysine, ornithine and arginine in the kidney and intestine. There is precipitation of cystine in the urine, with formation of crystals and calculi. Radiographically, cystine stones are radiopaque, with a smooth appearance, and less dense than calcium stones.

20. Syringomyelia ★★★★
    90% of syringomyelia cases are associated with Arnold–Chiari syndrome.

ANSWERS TO CASE HISTORIES

Case I

1. CSF examination ★★★★
   Brain biopsy ★★★★
   Electroencephalogram ★★★★
   VDRL TPHA ★★★★

2. Jakob-Creutzfeld disease ★★★★

Alzheimer's disease ★★
Multiple sclerosis ★★
Jakob-Creutzfeld disease is a slow, viral encephalopathy, resulting in a rapidly progressing dementia with myoclonus, extrapyramidal signs and the presence of multifocal cortical symptoms. The disease usually progresses to death within a few months. It is characterised by profound neuronal loss, astrocytosis, and a typical spongiform degeneration of the entire brain. Brain homogenates transmit the disease, in serial passages, to chimpanzees and guinea-pigs, while transmission to humans from corneal implants has also been noted, suggesting a viral aetiology.

Case II

1. Blood cultures ★★★★
   Vaginal swab and cytology ★★★★
   CT scan of the head ★★
   VDRL TPHA ★★
   Electron microscopy of CSF ★★
   Viral antibody titres (for herpes simplex) ★★
   Electroencephalogram ★★

2. Herpes simplex meningitis ★★★★
   Extradural abscess ★★
   Herpes simplex type I is associated with encephalitis, whereas type II is associated with aseptic meningitis, and occasionally with a polyradiculitis frequently in association with genital infection by the same strain. Radicular pain is often over lower lumbar and sacral dermatomes. The pain may mimic symptoms of a herniated intervertebral disc, but is often temporally associated with the eruptions of genital herpes. A further cause of back pain with this condition is the presence of lymphadenopathy in the pelvic and para-aortic lymph nodes.

Case III

1. Liver biopsy ★★★★
   Bromsulphalein excretion test ★★★★
   Ultrasound of liver ★★★★
   ERCP 0
   Cholecystogram 0

2. Dubin-Johnson syndrome ★★★★
   Cholestatic jaundice ★
   Acute hepatitis 0
   The Dubin-Johnson syndrome is a chronic benign, intermittent icterus, with conjugated hyperbilirubinaemia and bilirubinuria. Pruritus is absent, and serum alkaline phosphatase and bile acid levels are normal. In a prolonged bromsulphalein excretion test, after an initial fall in serum level the BSP rises so that the value at 120 minutes exceeds that at 45 minutes. The condition may present as jaundice during pregnancy, or after taking oral contraceptives, both of which reduce hepatic excretory function. Macroscopically, the liver is greenish-black, with dense melanin pigment in liver cells and Kupffer cells related to lysosomes on electron microscopy. The prognosis is excellent.

Case IV

1. Sputum cytology and culture ★★★★
   Barium swallow ★★★★
   Bronchoscopic biopsy in zone of consolidation ★★
   Gastric washings for acid-fast bacilli ★★
   CT scan of lungs ★★
   Lung function tests ★★

2. Lipoid pneumonia ★★★★
   Recurrent aspiration pneumonia due to diverticulum or achalasia ★★★★
   Bronchial carcinoma ★★★★
   Pulmonary tuberculosis ★★
   Bronchopneumonia ★★
   Aspiration of oil into the lungs may cause acute reactions such as haemorrhagic bronchopneumonia, with insidious reactions leading to lobar damage. Lipid is initially present in the alveolar

Answers

phagocytes, lying free in alveoli or collecting in the interstitium, in a peribronchiolar or subpleural location. There they evoke first a cellular and eventually a collagenous response, with lesions resembling those of liquid paraffin granulomas. The end-result is a diffuse interstitial fibrosis. There is usually absence of marked inflammatory reactions.

Case V

1. Paired renin and aldosterone estimations ★★★★
   Angiotensin infusion, for resistance to the pressor effect of angiotensin ★★★★
   Faecal phenolphthalein screen ★★★★
   Urinary electrolytes ★★★★

2. Barrter's syndrome ★★★★

ANSWERS TO DATA INTERPRETATIONS

1. Complete A-V dissociation ★★★★
   Left axis deviation ★★★★
   Incomplete right bundle branch block ★★★★
   U waves ★★★★

2. Cirrhosis of the liver ★★★★
   Hypoalbuminaemia and diffuse increase in the gamma globulin ★★★★
   Nephrotic syndrome 0
   The normal electrophoretic strip is made up of the following proteins: albumin, α_1 globulin, α_2 globulin, β globulin and γ globulin. The patient in **C** has a reduced albumin fraction and a diffusely increased globulin fraction, with near-fusion of the β-γ bands. Often in cirrhosis the α_1 is reduced.
   The α_1 fraction is made up of: α_1 antitrypsin
   α_1 glycoprotein
   α lipoprotein
   The α_2 fraction is made up of: α_2 macroglobulin
   haptoglobulin
   caeruloplasmin
   The β globulin is made up of: β lipoprotein
   transferrin
   complement
   The γ globulin contains all immunoglobulins.

3. (a) Tensilon test (edrophonium chloride test) ★★★★
   Plasma potassium ★★★★
   Serum calcium ★★★★
   Acetyl choline receptor antibodies ★★★★
   EMG ★★
   Chest X-ray ★★
   Antistriated muscle antibody ★★
   Screening of diaphragms ★
   Thyroxine ★
   (b) Alveolar hypoventilation ★★★★
   Respiratory muscle weakness ★★★★
   In myashemia gravis, weakness of skeletal muscle is characteristically increased by exercise and not associated with muscle pain. Ocular muscles are involved in 70% of cases, and bulbar muscle weakness leads to loss of facial expression, inability to whistle, difficulty with speech, chewing and swallowing. Respiratory muscle involvement (as in this case) leads to dyspnoea and ventilatory failure in severe cases. The disease is caused by acetyl choline receptor antibodies which reduce the number of receptors to typically about one-third. This reduction accounts for the reduction in amplitude of the end-plate potential, which may thus fail to trigger an action potential and hence muscle contraction.

4. (a) Barium swallow ★★★★
   Electromyography ★★★★
   Oesophagoscopy with biopsy ★★★★

   Needle biopsy of muscle ★★★★
   Blood gases ★★
   (b) Dermatomyositis ★★★★
   Dermatomyositis with oesophageal carcinoma ★★★★
   Myasthenia gravis 0
   Underlying malignancy is found in 5–8% of patients with dermatomyositis. Muscle aching and tenderness is experienced by 50% of patients. Muscle weakness is greatest proximally and is usually symmetrical, and atrophy is common. Bulbar muscle involvement produces dysphagia or dysphonia. Ocular muscle involvement is very rare. Respiratory muscle weakness is common. Muscle enzymes and biopsy are helpful diagnostically, as is electromyography which characteristically shows fibrillation, polyphasic action potentials, and occasionally bizarre, high frequency repetitive discharges.

5. (a) Small bowel enema ★★★★
   Jejunal biopsy ★★★★
   Stool culture for parasites (e.g. giardia cysts) ★★★★
   Red cell folate ★★★★
   Dietary history ★★★★
   B12 estimation ★
   (b) Folate deficiency, inducing macrocytic anaemia ★★★★
   B12 deficiency 0
   Normal deoxyuridine-induced suppression of ^3H thymidine uptake is restored on incubating folic acid with the patient's marrow, confirming the diagnosis of folic acid deficiency.
   Causes include:
   Nutritional;
   Malabsorption (e.g. tropical sprue, coeliac disease, partial gastrectomy);
   Excessive utilisation (e.g. pregnancy, lactation, haemolytic anaemia, myelosclerosis, carcinoma, myeloma, Crohn's disease, psoriasis, exfoliative dermatitis);
   Anticoagulant drug therapy, alcoholism, liver disease.

6. Left axis deviation ★★★★
   Anterolateral myocardial infarction ★★★★
   Right bundle branch block ★★★★
   Sinus bradycardia ★★★★

7. (a) Blood film ★★★★
   Dietary history ★★★★
   Small bowel enema ★★★★
   Jejunal biopsy ★★★★
   Red cell folate and B12 levels ★★★★
   Urinary calcium ★★
   Bone X-rays and biopsy ★★
   Fe and TIBC estimation ★★
   (b) Intestinal malabsorption ★★★★
   Dietary insufficiency ★★★★

8. (a) Drug-induced proximal tubulopathy ★★★★
   (b) Aminoglycoside therapy should be stopped ★★★★
   Potassium, calcium, magnesium and phosphate should be replaced ★★★★
   Aminoglycosides (AG) could precipitate this type of proximal tubular damage. AG are excreted virtually unchanged by the kidney, renal damage being dose-dependent, occurring typically in dehydrated patients or in those with impaired renal function. Because of their amino acid grouping, they are taken up by proximal tubular cells. With increasing tubular cell concentration of aminoglycoside, damage occurs producing the features of proximal tubulopathy. Other potential nephrotoxins in this context include cephalosporins, amphotericin B and tetracyclines.

9. (a) Gilbert's syndrome ★★★★
   (b) Diagnostic trial of phenobarbitone ★★★★
   24 hour 400kcal fast ★★★★
   Liver biopsy 0
   Bromsulphthalein retention 0

Gilbert's syndrome is the commonest form of familial, unconjugated, non-haemolytic hyperbilirubinaemia, affecting 2–5% of the population. It has an excellent prognosis. Jaundice is mild and intermittent, and deepening often follows intercurrent infection. There is associated malaise, nausea, and often discomfort over the liver. However, liver histology is normal. Several abnormalities are present: UDP glucuronyl transferase is reduced, and liver uptake of bilirubin may be defective. An increase in bilirubin follows a 24 hour 400kcal diet, probably due to an increase in serum fatty acid on fasting which competes with bilirubin for excretion by the liver cell. Phenobarbitone 60mg t.d.s. will return bilirubin to normal.

10. (a) Blood glucose ★★★★
       Urine and blood cultures ★★★★
       ECG ★★★★
       Chest X-ray ★★★★
       Cardiac enzymes ★★
    (b) Hyperosmolar hyperglycaemic coma (HHC) ★★★★
       HHC with urinary infection ★★★★
In hyperosmolar coma, the insulin resistance of ketoacidosis is usually absent. Treatment should be with isotonic saline and insulin. Hypotonic solutions should not be administered until the patient's volume is stabilised, and then only slowly and judiciously. Potassium repletion may be necessary.

Index

Abducent nerve palsy 5.5, 5.11
Abscesses
    brain 5.6, 5.11, 9.7, 9.11
    liver, pyogenic 10.6, 10.11
    peritonsillar 7.3, 7.10
    subdural 4.7, 4.11
Acanthosis nigricans 2.3, 2.10, 7.3, 7.9, 8.9, 8.12
Achalasia 6.5, 6.11
Achlorhydria 7.9, 7.12
Acidosis
    anion gap 7.9, 7.12
    hyperchloraemic 1.9, 1.12, 4.9, 4.12
    lactic 3.6, 3.11
    metabolic
        with metabolic alkalosis 2.9, 2.12
        methanol and 3.6, 3.11
        with mixed respiratory alkalosis 2.9, 2.12
    renal tubular 1.9, 1.12
Acquired immune deficiency syndrome, herpes genitalis 1.4, 1.10
Acromegaly 6.5, 6.11, 10.9, 10.12, 12.4, 12.11
Actinomycosis 3.3, 3.10
Acute intermittent porphyria 5.6, 5.11
Acute lymphoblastic leukaemia 4.3, 4.9, 4.10, 4.12, 11.10
    Conn's 4.2, 4.10, 5.6, 5.11
    pituitary 3.6, 3.11
Addison's disease 5.5, 5.11
Adenoma sebaceum 11.3, 11.10
Adrenal hyperplasia
    nodular 5.6, 5.11
    congenital 4.6, 4.11
Adrenocortical failure, secondary 7.9, 7.12
Air encephalogram 2.4, 2.10
Airways, obstruction 7.9, 7.12
Alcoholic liver disease 6.3, 6.10
Alkalosis
    metabolic, with metabolic acidosis 2.9, 2.12
    mixed respiratory, with, metabolic acidosis 2.9, 2.12
Alkaptonuria 7.2, 7.10, 11.2, 11.10
Alveolar hypoventilation 12.9, 12.12
Alveolitis, fibrosing 7.2, 7.10
Aminoglycosides 12.9, 12.12
Amiodarone therapy, thyroid function tests in 3.9, 3.12
Amyloidosis 1.2, 1.10, 5.9, 5.12
    cutaneous 9.2, 9.10
    renal 2.5, 2.11
Amyotrophy, bilateral neuralgic 2.7, 2.12
Anaemia
    autoimmune haemolytic 1.9, 1.12
    haemolytic 4.4, 4.10, 5.2
        Heinz body 10.9, 10.12
    iron deficiency 7.3, 7.5, 7.10, 7.11, 10.5, 10.11
        biochemical data 9.9, 9.12
    macrocytic 12.8, 12.12
    megaloblastic 8.5, 8.11
    sickle cell 5.10
Anaphylactoid purpura 3.2, 3.10
Androgen resistance, complete 10.4, 10.10
Androgen-secreting tumour 3.9, 3.12
Aneurysm, anterior communicating artery 6.2, 6.10
Angiodysplasia 7.7, 7.12
Angioid streaks, retina 3.4, 3.10
Angiokeratoma corporis diffusum 11.4, 11.10
Anion gap
    absence of 8.9, 8.12
    acidosis 7.9, 7.12
Anisocytosis 7.3, 7.10, 8.5, 8.11
Anti-diuretic hormone (ADH)
    abnormalities 9.9, 9.12
    disturbances 2.9, 2.12
Antibiotics and diarrhoea 8.6, 8.11
Aorta, dissection of 2.6, 2.11
Aortic
    regurgitation 1.9, 1.11, 11.9, 11.11
    stenosis 10.9, 10.12
Arachnodactyly, congenital contractual 2.4, 2.10
Arachnoid cyst 8.3, 8.10
Arcus senilis 10.5, 10.11
Argyrosis 4.3, 4.10, 7.4, 7.11
Arsenic poisoning 3.11
    squamous carcinomata in 3.5, 3.11
Arteriography, hypotension during 2.6, 2.11

Arteriovenous
    fistula/malformation 10.3, 10.10
    shunting, pulmonary 3.9, 3.12
Arteritis, giant cell 1.6, 1.10, 2.2, 2.10, 8.7, 8.12
Arthritis, gonococcal 2.9, 2.12
    mutilans 12.3, 12.10
    psoriatic 6.4, 6.10, 12.3, 12.10
    rheumatoid 3.2, 3.10, 5.5, 5.11, 6.3, 6.5, 6.10, 6.11, 9.2, 9.10
    septic 2.9, 2.12
Arthrochalasis multiplex congenita 6.4, 6.10
Asbestosis 9.4, 9.10
Ascaris infection 2.3, 2.10, 4.4, 4.10
Atrial
    fibrillation 10.8, 10.11
    flutter 8.8, 8.12
        with variable block 2.9, 2.12
    hypertrophy
        left 3.8, 3.9, 3.11, 3.12, 5.9, 5.12
    myxoma 8.6, 8.11
    septal defect 2.4, 2.10, 3.9, 3.12,10.7,10.11
Atrioventricular
    block 6.8, 6.12
    dissociation 12.8, 12.12
Autoimmune
    haemolytic anaemia 1.9, 1.12
    thrombocytopenia 4.9, 4.12
Axis deviation
    left 5.9, 5.12, 7.8, 7.12, 10.8, 10.11, 11.8, 11.11, 12.8, 12.9, 12.12
    right 3.9, 3.12

Bacterial endocarditis 6.3, 6.10
Balanitis circinata 8.3, 8.10
Barium follow-through 2.3, 2.10
Barrter's syndrome 12.7, 12.12
Bazin's disease 2.2, 2.10
Becker's dystrophy 11.5, 11.10
Behçet's disease 7.5, 7.11, 8.3, 8.10
Biceps tendon, ruptures 6.3, 6.10
Bigeminus rhythm 5.9, 5.12, 7.8, 7.12
Bilharzia 11.3, 11.10
Biliary sclerosis, primary 9.4, 9.10
Biliary tree, gas/barium in 4.1, 4.10
Bitot's spot 5.3, 5.10
Biventricular failure 10.7, 10.11
Boutonniere deformity 9.2, 9.10
Bowel
    inflammatory disease 8.3, 8.10
    tuberculous ulcers 4.4, 4.10
Bowen's disease 3.11
Bradycardia, sinus 12.9, 12.12
Brain
    abscess 5.6, 5.11, 9.7, 9.11
    damage, in systemic lupus erythematosus 7.6, 7.11
    extradural haematoma 1.5, 1.10
    haemorrhage 7.6–7, 7.11
    subdural abscess 4.7, 4.11
    supratentorial lesion 1.6, 1.10
    third ventricle
        calcification 1.3, 1.10
        colloid cyst 2.4, 2.10
    tumour 3.3, 3.10
Brainstem
    cerebrovascular accident 3.7, 3.11
    distortion 1.6, 1.10
    encephalitis 5.7, 5.12, 11.7, 11.11
    haemorrhage 5.7, 5.12, 7.6–7, 7.11
    infarction 5.7, 5.12
    oedema 5.7, 5.12
Bronchial carcinoma 1.7, 1.11
Bronchiectasis 7.2, 7.10, 9.9, 9.12
Brown–Sequard syndrome 9.6, 9.11
Brucellosis 6.6–7, 6.11
Brushfield spots 6.3, 6.10
Budd–Chiari syndrome 8.4, 8.11
Bullous pemphigoid 6.2, 6.10
Bundle branch block
    left 1.8, 1.11, 5.9, 5.12, 10.8, 10.11
    right 9.8, 9.12, 12.9, 12.12
    incomplete 2.8, 2.12, 3.9, 3.12, 5.8, 5.12, 12.8, 12.12

Caecum, carcinoma 9.4, 9.10
Calcification
    hilar lymph node 8.5, 8.11
    third ventricle 1.3, 1.10
Calyces, clubbing 7.2, 7.10
Candidiasis, oral 9.2, 9.10
Carcinoma
    bronchial 1.7, 1.11
    caecal 9.4, 9.10
    oat cell 10.2, 10.10
    oesophageal 12.8, 12.12
    papillary, of the thyroid 5.3, 5.10
    small cell 10.2, 10.10
    squamous, in arsenic poisoning 3.5, 3.11
Catecholamine-secreting tumour 2.2, 2.10
Cardiomyopathy, congestive 9.6, 9.11
Cerebellar
    haemorrhage 7.6–7, 7.11
    infarction 5.7, 5.12
    oedema 5.7, 5.12
Cerebral see brain
Cerebrovascular accident, brainstem 3.7, 3.11
Charcot–Marie–Tooth disease 1.3, 1.10
Chest, multiple cavitating lesions 2.2, 2.10
Chlamydial perihepatitis 5.7, 5.12
Cholelithiasis 4.4, 4.10
Choroid
    naevus 1.2, 1.10, 10.2, 10.10
    tubercle 2.2, 2.10
Chronic lymphocytic leukaemia 1.9, 1.12, 2.4, 2.11
Clofibrate therapy 1.9, 1.12
Coeliac disease 1.5, 1.10
Cold agglutination disease, blood in 3.2, 3.10
Cold haemagglutinin disease 6.9, 6.12
Colitis
    acute ulcerative 1.2, 1.10
    ischaemic 10.3, 10.10
Collagen disease 2.9, 2.12
Colloid cyst of third ventricle 2.4, 2.10
Coloboma of the eye 5.2, 5.10
Colon
    angiodysplasia 7.7, 7.12
    sigmoid, volvulus 1.3, 1.10
    toxic dilatation 8.6, 8.11
Coma, hyperosmolar hyperglycaemic 12.9, 12.13
Communicating artery, anterior, aneurysm 6.2, 6.10
Congestive cardiomyopathy 9.6, 9.11
Conjunctivitis, phlyctenular 2.10, 9.4, 9.10
Conn's adenoma 4.2, 4.10, 5.6, 5.11
Contraceptives, oral 1.9, 1.12
Cornea, keratic precipitates 11.4, 11.10
Coxsackie virus infection 11.4, 11.10
Cranial nerves, third, palsy 2.4, 2.10
Craniopharyngoma 1.3, 1.10
Cricopharyngeal web 7.5, 7.11
Crohn's disease 8.3, 8.10
    ocular manifestations 9.4, 9.10
    small intestine 4.2, 4.10
Cryoglobulinaemia 3.2, 3.10
Cushing's syndrome 5.9, 5.12
Cyanotic heart disease 7.2, 7.10, 9.9, 9.12
Cyclosporin therapy 12.2, 12.10
    effects of 1.2, 1.10
Cystic
    fibrosis 7.2, 7.10
    teratoma 7.4, 7.10
Cystine stones 12.4, 12.11
Cystinuria 12.11
Cytomegalovirus infection 2.9, 2.12, 8.9, 8.12, 10.9, 10.12
    blood in 3.2, 3.10

Darier's sign 7.10
Dermatitis, contagious pustular 8.4, 8.10
Dermatomyositis 6.4, 6.10, 9.2, 9.10, 12.2, 12.8, 12.10, 12.12
    with oesophageal carcinoma 12.8, 12.12
Dermoid cyst 7.4, 7.10
Diabetes insipidus, nephrogenic 11.9, 11.11
Diabetes mellitus
    dermopathy 10.4, 10.10

    insulin-resistant 8.9, 8.12
Diaphragmatic weakness 10.7, 10.11
Diarrhoea, antibiotic-related 8.6, 8.11
Diazoxide therapy 12.3, 12.10
Dietary insufficiency 12.9, 12.12
Diphtheria 4.3, 4.10
Disseminated intravascular coagulation 9.9, 9.12
Dopamine antagonists 8.2, 8.10
Down's syndrome, ocular manifestations 6.3, 6.10
Dressler's syndrome 11.5, 11.10
Drugs
    fixed eruption 1.4, 1.10
    overdose, tricyclic antidepressants 1.7, 1.11
Dubin–Johnson syndrome 12.6, 12.11
Duodenal
    folds, thickening 2.5, 2.11
    ulceration with scarring 10.4, 10.10
Dupuytren's contracture 3.2, 3.10

Ear, relapsing polychondritis 5.3, 5.10
Echocardiograms, interpretation 1.9, 1.11
Ehlers–Danlos syndrome 6.4, 6.10, 8.5, 8.11, 12.4, 12.10
Elliptocytosis 5.2, 5.10
Emphysema 7.9, 7.12
Empyema necessitans 4.5, 4.11
Encephalitis
    brainstem 5.7, 5.12, 11.7, 11.11
    herpes simplex 5.6, 5.11
    viral 11.7, 11.11
Encephalography, air 2.4, 2.10
Endocarditis, subacute bacterial 6.3, 6.10, 12.2, 12.10
Enterocolitis, staphylococcal 8.6, 8.11
Epidermal necrolysis, toxic 11.6, 11.11
Epidermolysis bullosa dystrophica 5.5, 5.11
Epiloica 11.4, 11.10
Erythema
    contagiosum 8.4, 8.10
    gyratum repens 7.3, 7.10
    induratum 2.2, 2.10
    marginatum 4.2, 4.10
Eye, superior oblique palsy 3.5, 3.10

Fabry's disease 11.5, 11.10
Feet, neuropathic 12.2, 12.10
Felty's syndrome 8.10–11
Femoral neck, pseudofracture 12.3, 12.10
Fibroma, periungual 11.4, 11.10
Fibrosing alveolitis 7.2, 7.10
Fitz-Hugh–Curtis syndrome 5.7, 5.12
Folate (folic acid) deficiency 8.5, 8.11, 9.3, 9.10, 12.8, 12.12
Friedreich's ataxia 1.3, 1.10
Fructose intolerance 3.9, 3.12

Gall stones 5.2
    in common bile duct 12.4, 12.10
Gastric folds, thickening 2.5, 2.11
Gastric lymphoma 3.5, 3.10
Gaucher's disease 4.6–7, 4.11, 8.10–11, 10.2, 10.10
Giant cell
    arteritis 1.6, 1.10, 8.7, 8.12
    tumour 11.4, 11.10
Giardiasis with malabsorption 8.9, 8.12
Gilbert's syndrome 12.9, 12.12–13
Gingiva
    fibromatosis, familial 3.2, 3.10
    hyperplasia 1.2, 1.10
Glaucoma 11.4, 11.10
    acute closed angle 7.4, 7.10
    rubeotic 3.5, 3.10
    simplex, chronic 11.4, 11.10
Glomerulonephritis
    acute 10.7, 10.11
    focal 6.9, 6.12
Glycogen storage disease 11.9, 11.12
Gonadal dysgenesis 9.9, 9.12
Gonococcal arthritis 2.9, 2.12
    septicaemia 10.4, 10.10

Index

Goodpasture's syndrome 3.9, 3.12
Gout 1.4, 1.10
Gouty tophus 11.10, 11.12
Granuloma
    annulare 11.4, 11.10
    non-caseating 5.10
Granulomatosis, Wegener's 6.6, 6.11
    ocular manifestations 9.7, 9.11
Graves' disease 5.3, 10.2, 10.10
    ophthalmopathy 1.5, 1.10
Guillain–Barré syndrome 11.7, 11.11
    papilloedema in 4.2, 4.10

Haematoma
    extradural 1.5, 1.10
    subdural 1.6, 1.10
Haemochromatosis with cirrhosis 8.2, 11.10
Haemolytic anaemia 4.4, 4.10, 5.3, 5.10
    autoimmune 1.9, 1.12
    Heinz body 10.9, 10.12
    uraemic syndrome 6.9, 6.12
Haemoptysis 5.3, 5.10
Haemosiderosis, transfusion 3.9, 3.12
Hair, perifollicular haemorrhage 3.2, 3.10
Hands, ulnar deviation 6.5, 6.11
Head injury, biochemical data 2.9, 2.12
Heart block
    complete 4.8, 4.11
        with ventricular escape 10.9, 10.12
    first degree 7.8, 7.12
Heart disease, cyanotic 7.2, 7.10, 9.9, 9.12
Heart failure, hypertensive 10.7, 10.11
Heinz body haemolytic anaemia 10.9, 10.12
Hemiblock, left anterior 2.8, 2.12, 7.8, 7.12
Henoch–Schönlein purpura 3.2, 3.10
Hepatitis 1.9, 1.12
    chronic active 12.5, 12.11
Hepatoma, erythropoietin-secreting 3.9, 3.12
Hereditary haemorrhagic telangiectasia 5.3, 5.10
Heredity
    autosomal recessive 11.8, 11.11
    X-linked recessive 8.9, 8.12
    X-linked trait 4.9, 4.12
Heroin abuse 10.9, 10.12
Herpes genitalis 1.4, 1.10, 5.3, 5.10
Herpes gestationis 12.2, 12.10
Herpes simplex
    encephalitis 5.6, 5.11
    infection 1.4, 1.10, 5.3, 5.10
    meningitis 12.6, 12.11
Herpes zoster infection 12.5, 12.11
Hilar lymph node calcification 8.5, 8.11
Histiocytosis X 10.5, 10.11
Homocystinuria 6.4, 6.10
Hurler's syndrome 1.4, 1.10
Hydrocephalus 1.3, 1.10
    cerebellar infarction 5.7, 5.12
Hyperaldosteronism 4.9, 4.12, 5.6, 5.9, 5.11, 5.12
Hypercalcaemia 4.4, 4.10, 9.9, 9.12
    malignancy associated 11.9, 11.12
Hyperchloraemic acidosis 1.4, 1.12, 4.9, 4.12
Hyperkalaemia ECG 4.8, 4.11
Hyperlipidaemia 1.2, 1.10, 8.2, 8.10, 10.5, 10.11
Hypernephroma 4.3, 4.10
Hyperosmolar hyperglycaemic coma 12.9, 12.13
Hyperparathyroidism, primary 2.6, 2.11, 7.8, 7.11
Hyperprolactinaemia 8.2, 8.10
Hypertension, malignant, papilloedema in 4.2 ,4.10
Hypertrichosislanuginosa 12.3, 12.10
Hypertriglyceridaemia 9.10
Hypertrophic obstructive cardiomyopathy, ECG 3.8, 3.11
Hypertrophy
    atrial 3.8, 3.9, 3.11, 3.12, 5.9, 5.12
    septal 3.8, 3.11
    ventricular 3.8, 3.11
Hypervitaminosis A 7.6, 7.10
Hypervitaminosis D 11.9, 11.12
Hypoalbuminaemia 12.8, 12.12
Hypocalcaemia, ECG 8.8, 8.12

Hypochromia 7.3, 7.10
Hypoglycaemia, reactive 4.9, 4.12
Hypomagnesaemia, ECG 8.8, 8.12
Hypotension during arteriography 2.6, 2.11
Hypothyroidism 2.9, 2.12, 11.9 ,11.12
    primary 8.2, 8.10
Hypoventilation, alveolar 12.8, 12.12

Ileum, tuberculous ulcers 4.4, 4.10
Impetigo contagiosum 8.2, 8.10
Infection, chronic 10.5, 10.11
Infectious mononucleosis 1.9, 1.12, 4.3, 4.10, 8.9, 8.12
    blood in 3.2, 3.10
Inflammatory bowel disease 8.3, 8.10
Inheritance see heredity
Injection sites, infected, drug addicts 7.2, 7.10
Insulin resistance 8.9, 8.12
Insulinoma 2.6, 2.11
Interphalangeal joints
    proximal, swelling 1.4, 1.10
    valgus deformity 6.5, 6.11
Intestinal malabsorption 12.9, 12.12
Intracranial pressure, raised, papilloedema in 4.2, 4.10
Iron deficiency anaemia 5.3, 5.10, 7.3, 7.5, 7.9, 7.10, 10.5, 10.11
    biochemical data 9.9, 9.12
Ischaemia, subendocardial 8.8, 8.12

Jakob–Creutzfeld disease 12.6, 12.11
Janeway lesion 12.2, 12.10
Jervell–Lange–Nielsen syndrome 8.8, 8.12
Joid–Basedow effect 3.12

Kala-azar 12.4, 12.10
Kaposi's sarcoma 7.5, 7.11
Kayser–Fleischer rings 6.3, 6.10
Keratoconjunctivitis, phlyctenular 2.10, 9.4, 9.10
Keratoderma, palmoplantar 6.2, 6.10
Kidneys
    adult polycystic 7.12
    medullary sponge 9.5, 9.10
    see also renal
Knee joint, effusions 5.5, 5.11
Lactic acidosis 3.6, 3.11
Lag storage curve 4.9, 4.12
Laser therapy 1.4, 1.10
LE cell phenomenon 12.5, 12.11
Lead poisoning 8.2, 8.10
Leishmaniasis 12.3, 12.10
    visceral 9.6, 9.11
Leprosy 1.3, 1.10, 8.3, 8.10
    tuberculoid 8.7, 8.11
Leptospirosis 1.6–7, 1.11
Leser–Trélat syndrome 1.5, 1.10
Leukaemia
    acute lymphoblastic 4.3, 4.9, 4.10 ,4.12, 11.3, 11.10
    chronic lymphocytic 1.9, 1.12, 2.4, 2.11
Leukaemoid reaction 8.9, 8.12
Leydig tumour of testis 2.2, 2.10
Lichen planus 12.2, 12.10
Limb girdle dystrophy 10.5, 10.10
Lingual thyroid 3.2, 3.10
Lipaemia retinalis 5.2, 5.10
Lipoid pneumonia 12.7, 12.11
Liver
    abscess, pyogenic 10.6, 10.11
    chronic disease 10.4, 10.11
    cirrhosis
        alcoholic 6.3, 6.10
        with erythropoietin secreting hepatoma 3.9, 3.12
        with secondary polycthaemia 3.9, 3.12
Looser's zone 12.3, 12.10
Lung defect, restrictive 4.9, 4.12
Lungs, honey-combing 10.5, 10.11
Lupus vulgaris 7.3, 7.10
Lymphatic leukaemia 2.4, 2.11
Lymymphoblastic leukaemia 4.3, 4.9, 4.10, 4.12, 11.3, 11.10
Lymphocytic leukaemia 1.9, 1.12

Lymphoma
    blood in 3.2, 3.10
    cutaneous 4.4, 4.10
    gastric 3.5, 3.10
    non-Hodgkin's 11.9, 11.11

Macrocytes, oval 8.5, 8.11
Macrocytic anaemia 12.8, 12.12
Malabsorption 5.9, 5.12, 10.9, 10.12
    giardiasis and 8.9, 8.12
    intestinal 12.9, 12.12
    pancreatic 4.9, 4.12
Malaria 2.4, 2.11, 9.5, 9.11
Malignancy 9.9, 9.12
    occult 8.7, 8.12
Malignant melanoma 7.5, 7.11
Mallory bodies 6.3, 6.10
Marfan's syndrome 2.4, 2.10, 6.4, 6.10, 7.12
Mastocytosis 7.3, 7.10
Mee's lines 3.11
Megaloblastic anaemia 8.5, 8.11
Melanoma, malignant 7.5, 7.11
Meningioma 3.3, 3.10
    frontal 4.5, 4.11
Meningitis, herpetic 12.6, 12.11
Metabolic
    acidosis see acidosis, metabolic
    alkalosis see alkalosis, metabolic
    myopathy 10.5, 10.10
Metacarpophalangeal joints, valgus deformity 6.5, 6.11
Metatarsophalangeal joints, valgus deformity 6.5, 6.11
Methanol consumption and metabolic acidosis 3.6, 3.11
    microcytosis 7.2, 7.9
MIBI/technetium subtraction scan 11.1, 11.10
Midbrain, haemorrhage 1.6, 1.10
Milk alkali syndrome 9.9, 9.12
Minoxidil therapy 12.3, 12.10
Mitral valves
    echocardiograms 1.9, 1.11
    incompetence 10.8, 10.11
    prolapse 1.11
    prosthesis, complications of 6.6. 6.11
    stenosis 1.9, 1.11, 10.8, 10.11
Molluscum contagiosum 11.4, 11.10
Moniliasis, oesophageal 11.5, 11.11
Morphoea 11.3, 11.10
Moschkovitz syndrome 2.9, 2.12
Motor neurone disease 10.5, 10.11
MRI scan, gallium-enhanced 2.2, 2.10
Multiple sclerosis 2.7, 2.12, 3.7, 3.11
Myasthenia gravis 6.9, 6.12, 10.6–7, 10.11, 12.8, 12.12
Mycoplasma pneumonia, blood in 3.2, 3.10
Mycosis fungoides 4.4, 4.10
Myelitis, transverse 3.7, 3.11
Myelofibrosis 8.10–11
Myelogram, water-soluble 5.4, 5.10
Myeloma 1.9, 1.12, 3.8, 3.11, 10.5, 10.11
    multiple 3.3, 3.10
Myocardial infarction 3.6, 3.11, 5.9, 5.12, 11.8, 11.11
    anterior 7.8, 7.12
    anterolateral 12.9, 12.12
        acute 9.8, 9.12
    anteroseptal, acute 11.8, 11.11
    echocardiogram 1.5, 1.10
    inferior, acute 4.8, 4.11
Myopathy, metabolic 10.5, 10.10
Myxoma, atrial 1.9, 1.11, 4.3, 4.10, 8.6, 8.11

Naevus, choroid 1.2, 1.10, 10.2, 10.10
Necrobiosis lipoidica 9.3, 9.10
Necrotising vasculitis 7.3, 7.10
Nephrogenic diabetes insipidus 11.9, 11.11
Nephrotic syndrome 6.9, 6.12, 8.2, 8.10
Neurofibromatosis 5.5, 5.11, 9.2, 11.5, 11.11
Neuropathic ulcer 8.2, 8.10
Neurosyphilis 5.12
    parenchymatous 5.9, 5.12
Niacin deficiency 5.3, 5.10

Oat cell carcinoma 10.2, 10.10
Oesophageal
    carcinoma 12.8, 12.12
    moniliasis 11.5, 11.11
Onycholysis 6.4, 6.10
Ophthalmopathy
    Graves' 1.5, 1.10
    thyroid-associated 1.5, 1.10
Opiate narcosis 6.9, 6.12
Optic atrophy, negroid fundus 7.2, 7.10
Orf 8.4, 8.10
Osteogenesis imperfecta 10.5, 10.11
    tarda 5.5, 5.11
Osteomyelitis, pyogenic 11.6–7, 11.11
Osteoporosis, periarticular 6.5, 6.11
Otosclerosis 2.8, 2.12
Ovalocytosis 5.2, 5.10, 8.5, 8.11
Ovarian failure, premature 6.9, 6.12

Paget's disease 1.2, 1.10, 5.9, 5.12, 9.4, 9.10
Palmoplantar hyperkeratosis 6.2, 6.10
Pancreas malabsorption 4.9, 4.12
    neoplasm 6.4, 6.11
Pancreatitis, chronic 4.9, 4.12
Panphotocoagulation therapy 1.4, 1.10
Papilloedema 4.2, 4.10, 8.2, 8.10
Papyraceous scars on knee 8.5, 8.11
Paraganglioma, metastatic 2.2, 2.10
Paraneoplastic syndrome 1.7, 1.11
Paraproteinaemia 3.8, 3.11, 8.2, 8.9, 8.10, 8.12
Paraspinous ligament calcification 10.4, 10.10
Parathyroid adenoma 11.1, 1.10
Parenchymatous neurosyphilis 5.9, 5.12
Patterson–Kelly syndrome 7.11
Pellagra 5.3, 5.10
Pemphigoid, bullous 6.2, 6.10
Pencil cells 7.3, 7.10
Penicillin, skin eruptions 1.4, 1.10
Penis, balanitis circinata 8.3, 8.10
Penile pupillae 8.3, 8.10
Pentolinium test 5.9, 5.12
Pericardial disease 1.3, 1.10
Perifollicular haemorrhage 3.2, 3.10
Perihepatitis, chlamydial 5.7, 5.12
Peritoneal tuberculosis 4.7, 4.11
Periungual fibroma 11.4, 11.10
Peutz–Jeghers syndrome 3.5, 3.10
Phaeochromocytoma 2.2, 2.5, 2.10, 2.11, 11.6, 11.11
Pharyngitis, streptococcal 4.3, 4.10
Phenolphthalein, skin eruptions 1.4, 1.10
Phenothiazine 1.9, 1.12
Phenytoin, effects of 1.2, 1.10
Phlyctenular conjunctivitis 9.4, 9.10
Pingueculae 10.2, 10.10
Pituitary adenoma 2.2, 2.10, 3.6, 3.11, 5.4, 5.10
Plasmacytosis, reactive 10.4, 10.11
Plasmodium falciparum malaria 2.4, 2.11
Plasmodium vivax malaria 9.5, 9.11
Platelet defect, qualitative 5.9, 5.12
Plummer–Vinson syndrome 7.11
Pneumocystis carinii cysts 6.4, 6.10
Pneumonia
    lipoid 12.7, 12.11
    recurrent aspiration 12.7, 12.11
Pneumothorax 3.9, 3.12
    left apical 8.5. 8.11
Poikilocytosis 7.2, 7.9
Poliomyelitis 1.3, 1.10
Polyarteritis nodosa 6.3, 6.10, 7.3, 7.10, 12.2, 12.10
    ocular manifestations 9.6, 9.11
Polychondritis of ear 5.3, 5.10
Polycythaemia 3.9, 3.12
Polycythaemia rubra vera 9.2, 9.10, 11.9, 11.12
Polymyalgia rheumatica 8.7, 8.12
Polymyositis 10.4, 10.11
Polyneuritis, acute infective 11.7, 11.11
Porphyria
    acute intermittent 5.6, 5.11
    variegate 4.5, 4.11

Index

Pregnancy, biochemical data 1.9, 1.12
Presbyacusis 9.8, 9.12
Prolactinoma 3.6, 3.11, 8.2, 8.10
Protein-losing state 6.9, 6.12
Pseudofracture, femoral neck 12.3, 12.10
Pseudogout 2.5, 2.11, 10.9, 10.12
Pseudoxanthoma elasticum 6.4, 6.11
Psoriatic arthropathy 3.2, 3.10, 12.4, 12.10
Pulmonary
    A–V shunting 3.9, 3.12
    arteriogram 7.3, 7.10
    arteriovenous fistulae 5.3, 5.10
    embolus 3.9, 3.12, 7.3, 7.9, 7.10, 7.12
    infarct 7.5, 7.10
    oedema 3.6, 3.11, 7.9, 7.12
    tuberculosis 5.4, 5.10
Purpura
    anaphylactoid 3.2, 3.10
    Henoch–Schönlein 3.2, 3.10
    periorbital 1.2, 1.10
    thrombocytopenic 4.9, 4.12
    thrombotic thrombocytopenic 2.9, 2.12
Pyelonephritis, chronic 7.2, 7.10
Pyloric stenosis 7.9, 7.12
Pyoderma gangrenosum 2.3, 2.10, 6.3, 6.10
    bullous 3.2, 3.10
Pyrophosphate arthropathy 10.9, 10.12
    with synovitis 2.5, 2.11

Q waves 3.8, 3.11
QRS complexes, small 11.9, 11.11
QT interval prolongation 8.8, 8.12
Quinsy 7.3, 7.9–10

Refsum's disease 1.3, 1.10
Reiter's syndrome 8.3, 8.10
Renal
    amyloidosis 2.5, 2.11
    arteries
        occlusion 2.6, 2.11
        stenosis 12.4, 12.10
    failure 10.9, 10.12
        chronic 2.9, 2.12
    tubes, drug-induced damage 12.9, 12.12
    vein, thrombosis 6.9, 6.12
Rendu–Osler–Weber syndrome 5.3, 5.10
Respiratory function, restrictive 9.9, 9.12
Respiratory muscle weakness 12.8, 12.12
Retina, angioid streaks 3.3, 3.10
Retinal
    artery, branch occlusion 1.5, 1.10
    vein
        branch, occlusion 9.2, 9.10
        central, occlusion 8.2, 8.10
Retinoblastoma 4.3, 4.10
Rheumatic fever 4.2, 4.10
Rheumatoid arthritis 3.2, 3.10, 5.5, 5.11, 6.3, 6.5, 6.10, 6.11, 9.2, 9.10
    juvenile 4.4, 4.10
Rheumatoid joint, acute 2.9, 2.12
Rickets 10.2, 10.10
Romano–Ward syndrome 8.8, 8.12
Roth's spots 11.4, 11.10
Rubella immunity testing 8.9, 8.12

Sacroiliitis 10.4, 10.10
Sagittal vein thrombosis 6.7, 6.11
Salicylate
    consumption 1.9, 1.12
    Intoxication 1.9, 1.12
    poisoning 6.9, 6.12
Sarcoidosis 3.6–7, 3.11, 5.10, 7.5, 7.11, 8.3, 8.10, 9.9, 9.12, 11.9, 11.12
    cornea 11.4, 11.10
    cutaneous 7.2, 7.9, 9.4, 9.10, 12.2, 12.10
SBE with septic embolus 8.6, 8.11
Schistosoma mansoni 11.3, 11.10
Sclerae, blue 10.5, 10.11
Scleromalacia 12.2, 12.10

Sclerosis, systemic 6.5, 6.10, 10.5, 10.11
Scurvy 3.2, 3.10, 5.9, 5.12
'Sea fan' new vessel formation 6.2, 6.10
Septal hypertrophy 3.8, 3.11
Septicaemia, gonococcal 10.4, 10.10
Serratus anterior weakness 12.5, 12.11
Shoulder joint, effusion in 3.2, 3.10
Sickle cell disease 5.10
    ocular abnormalities 6.2, 6.10
Sigmoid volvulus 1.3, 1.10
Sinus
    arrest 6.8, 6.12
    bradycardia 12.9, 12.12
Skull, lytic lesions 10.5, 10.11
Spinal cord compression 9.6, 9.11
    by tumour 6.7, 6.11
Spine
    bamboo 10.4, 10.10
    gamma radioisotope image 1.4, 1.10
    metastatic cancer 5.2, 5.10
    neurofibromatosis 11.5, 11.11
    tumour, intramedullary 2.7, 2.12
Spleen
    indications for removal 8.4, 8.10–11
    infarct 7.6, 7.11
Sporotrichosis 7.2, 7.10
Staphylococcal enterocolitis 8.6, 8.11
Stevens–Johnson syndrome 6.2, 6.10
Still's disease 3.2, 3.10, 4.2, 4.4, 4.10
    cornea 11.4, 11.10
Stones
    common bile duct 12.4, 12.10
    cystine 12.4, 12.11
    see also gall stones
Streptococcal pharyngitis 4.3, 4.10
Stroke in evolution 8.7, 8.12
Strongyloidiasis 2.6–7, 2.11
Sturge–Weber syndrome 12.2, 12.10
Subdural
    abscess 4.7, 4.11
    haematoma 1.6, 1.10
Subendocardial
    changes, ECG 1.8, 1.11
    ischaemia 8.8, 8.12
Sulphasalazine treatment and haemolytic anaemia 10.9, 10.12
Sulphonamides
    allergic reaction 11.6, 11.11
    skin eruptions 1.4, 1.10
Synovitis pyrophosphate 2.5, 2.11
Syphilis
    congenital 7.5, 7.11
    cornea 11.4, 11.10
    late congenital 5.4, 5.10
    secondary 9.5, 9.11, 10.2, 10.9, 10.10, 10.12
    stigmata 5.10
    see also neurosyphilis
Syringomyelia 2.7, 2.12, 6.4, 6.11, 12.5, 12.11
Systemic lupus erythematosus 6.3, 6.10, 8.2, 8.10, 12.5, 12.11, 12.12
    biochemical data 2.9, 2.12, 10.9, 10.12
    cerebral 7.6, 7.11

T waves, low amplitude 11.9, 11.11
Tachycardia
    sinus 11.9, 11.11
    ventricular 7.8, 7.12
Target cells 7.3, 7.10
TBG excess 1.9, 1.12
Teeth, tetracycline staining 8.4, 8.11
Telangiectasia, hereditary haemorrhagic 5.3, 5.10
Teratoma, cystic 7.4, 7.10
Testicular feminization 10.4, 10.10
Testis, Leydig tumour 2.2, 2.10
Tetracycline staining of teeth 8.4, 8.11
Thalassaemia major 9.3, 9.10
Thost–Unna syndrome 6.2, 6.10
Thrombocythaemia, essential 9.12
Thrombocytopenia 8.5, 8.11, 10.3, 10.10
    autoimmune 4.9, 4.12
Thrombocytopenic purpura 4.9, 4.12

Thrombosis
    renal vein 6.9, 6.12
    sagittal vein 6.7, 6.11
    secondary causes 9.12
Thrombotic thrombocytopenic purpura 2.9, 2.12
Thyroid
    lingual 3.2, 3.10
    papillary carcinoma 5.3, 5.10
Thyroid crisis 10.6, 10.11
Thyroid function tests, amiodarone therapy 3.9, 3.12
Thyrotoxicosis 2.2, 2.10, 4.9, 4.12, 6.4, 6.10, 9.9, 9.12, 11.9, 11.12
    amiodarone therapy 3.9, 3.12
Tophus 1.4, 1.10, 11.3, 11.10
Toxocara infection 10.3, 10.10
    congenital 7.5, 7.11
Toxoplasmosis 2.9, 2.12, 8.9, 8.12
    congenital 7.5, 7.11
Transfusion haemosiderosis 3.9, 3.12
Tricyclic antidepressants, overdose 1.7, 1.11
Tuberculosis 3.6–7, 3.11
    cutaneous 7.10
    ileal ulcers 4.4, 4.10
    of the kidney 3.3, 3.10
    ocular 2.2, 2.10
    peritoneal 4.7, 4.11
Tumour
    giant cell 11.3, 11.10
    intracardiac 4.3, 4.10
    occult 8.7, 8.12
Turner's syndrome 9.9, 9.12
Tylosis 6.2, 6.10, 11.3, 11.10

U waves 12.8, 12.12
Ulcers
    duodenal, with scarring 10.4, 10.10
    neuropathic 8.2, 8.10
Ulnar nerve lesion 8.2, 8.10
Urticaria pigmentosa 7.3, 7.10

Valgus deformity 6.5, 6.11

Vasculitis
    allergic 3.2, 3.10
    necrotising 7.3, 7.10
    orbital 9.7, 9.11
Vena caval obstruction, inferior 8.5, 8.11
Ventilatory defect, restrictive 9.9, 9.12
Ventricle, third
    calcification 1.3, 1.10
    colloid cyst 2.4, 2.10
Ventricular
    demand pacemaker 5.8, 5.12
    fibrillation 7.8, 7.12
    hypertrophy, left 3.8, 3.11
    premature beats 1.8, 1.11, 6.8, 6.12
        with compensatory pulse 9.8, 9.12
            multiple multifocal 10.8, 10.11
    septal defect 3.5, 3.10
    tachycardia 7.8, 7.12
Vertebral artery
    dissection 3.7, 3.11
    embolism 3.7, 3.11
Virus infections 10.9, 10.12
Vision, left directional preponderance 5.8, 5.12
Vitamin A deficiency 5.3, 5.10
Vitamin A intoxication 7.7, 7.11
Vitamin B12 deficiency 8.5, 8.11, 9.3, 9.10
Vitamin D intoxication 9.9, 9.12, 11.9, 11.12
Von Willebrand's disease 7.12

Water intoxication 8.9, 8.12
Wegener's granulomatosis 6.6, 6.11
    ocular manifestations 9.7, 9.11
Wernicke's encephalopathy 4.6, 4.11
Wilson's disease 10.9, 10.12

Xanthelasmata 1.2, 1.10
Xanthomas, eruptive 9.3, 9.10

Zollinger–Ellison syndrome 2.5, 2.11